高等院校选用教材

免疫学双语实验技术指导
（第二版）

Current Protocols in Immunology A Laboratory Technology in Chinese and English Bilinguals

主编　章晓联

Editor-in-chief　Zhang Xiaolian

科学出版社

北京

内 容 简 介

　　本书是国内外第一本正式出版的医学免疫学双语(中文、英文)实验技术教学指导书籍,在初版的基础上内容更加丰富,既介绍了医学免疫学中的一些经典、传统的实验内容,又增添了目前使用的先进的实验技术(如各种免疫细胞纯化技术、糖免疫技术、肠道、肺部免疫细胞获取、流式细胞仪的多种检测方法应用等)。书中的每项实验包括实验原理、应用、材料、方法、结果、注意事项及思考题等。

　　本书适用于高等院校学生、教师,以及研究人员学习、参考、借鉴。

图书在版编目(CIP)数据

免疫学双语实验技术指导=Current Protocols in
Immunology A Laboratory Technology in Chinese and
English Bilinguals：汉、英/章晓联主编.—2 版.
—北京：科学出版社,2019.8
　　高等院校选用教材
　　ISBN 978 - 7 - 03 - 060363 - 0

　　Ⅰ.①免… Ⅱ.①章… Ⅲ.①免疫学—实验—高等学校—教学参考资料—汉、英 Ⅳ.①R392 - 33

中国版本图书馆 CIP 数据核字(2019)第 002875 号

责任编辑：朱　灵/责任校对：谭宏宇
责任印制：黄晓鸣/封面设计：殷　靓

科学出版社 出版
北京东黄城根北街 16 号
邮政编码：100717
http://www.sciencep.com

南京展望文化发展有限公司排版
广东虎彩云印刷有限公司印刷
科学出版社发行　各地新华书店经销

＊

2004 年 1 月第　一　版　开本：(787×1092) 1/16
2019 年 8 月第　二　版　印张：20 1/2
2024 年 1 月第八次印刷　字数：471 000

定价：65.00 元
(如有印装质量问题,我社负责调换)

《免疫学双语实验技术指导》(第二版)
编委会

潘 璆（武汉大学基础医学院）

邱文洪（江汉大学基础医学院）

屈子璐（武汉大学基础医学院）

史君宇（华中科技大学同济医学院）

苏 莉（华中科技大学生命科学与技术学院）

田野平（海军军医大学基础医学院）

王 瑾（武汉大学基础医学院）

吴 剑（武汉大学基础医学院）

吴雄文（华中科技大学同济医学院）

郗雪艳（湖北医药学院基础医学院）

向 田（恩施土家族苗族自治州中心医院）

肖 凌（湖北中医药大学检验学院）

谢 焱（武汉大学基础医学院）

姚琪利（武汉大学基础医学院）

尹丙姣（华中科技大学同济医学院）

曾凡帆（华中科技大学同济医学院）

曾瑞红（河北医科大学基础医学院）

张秋萍（武汉大学基础医学院）

章晓联（武汉大学基础医学院）

赵颖岚（南方科技大学）

郑 芳（华中科技大学同济医学院）

周永芹（三峡大学医学院）

周媛媛（武汉大学基础医学院）

Current Protocols in Immunology A Laboratory Technology in Chinese and English Bilinguals Editoral Board

Pan Qiu (School of Basic Medical Sciences, Wuhan University)

Qiu Wenhong (School of Basic Medical Sciences, Jianghan University)

Qu Zilu (School of Basic Medical Sciences, Wuhan University)

Shi Junyu (Tongji Medical College, Huazhong University of Science and Technology)

Su Li (College of Life Science & Technology, Huazhong University of Science and Technology)

Tian Yeping (School of Basic Medical Sciences, The Second Military Medical University)

Wang Jin (School of Basic Medical Sciences, Wuhan University)

Wu Jian (School of Basic Medical Sciences, Wuhan University)

Wu Xiongwen (Tongji Medical College, Huazhong University of Science and Technology)

Xi Xueyan (School of Basic Medical Sciences, Hubei University of Medicine)

Xiang Tian (The Central Hospital of Enshi Tujia and Miao Autonomous Prefecture)

Xiao Ling (School of Laboratory Medicine, Hubei University of Chinese Medicine)

Xie Yan (School of Basic Medical Sciences, Wuhan University)

Yao Qili (School of Basic Medical Sciences, Wuhan University)

Yin Bingjiao (Tongji Medical College, Huazhong University of Science and Technology)

Zeng Fanfan (Tongji Medical College, Huazhong University of Science and Technology)

Zeng Ruihong (School of Basic Medical Sciences, Hebei Medical University)

Zhang Qiuping (School of Basic Medical Sciences, Wuhan University)

Zhang Xiaolian (School of Basic Medical Sciences, Wuhan University)

Zhao Yinglan (Southern University of Science and Technology)

Zheng Fang (Tongji Medical College, Huazhong University of Science and Technology)

Zhou Yongqin (Medical College, China Three Gorges University)

Zhou Yuanyuan (School of Basic Medical Sciences, Wuhan University)

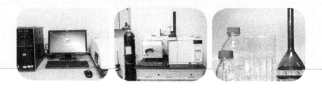

前 言

  《免疫学双语实验技术指导》是一本供高等院校大学生、研究生及教师使用和参考的免疫学双语教学实验技术指导教材。为了适应中国教学与国际教学接轨,高等院校普及双语教学的需要,编者在总结多年的实验教学经验的基础上,组织多名既具有出国留学经历,有很好的英语基础和英语能力的博士,又同时在第一线教学中具备丰富的医学免疫学教学经验的教授们,编写了这本免疫学双语教学实验技术指导。本书中英文对照,完全满足双语教学的需要,既是一本高等院校学生及教师急需的教材和参考书,也是国内外第一本正式出版的医学免疫学双语(中文、英文)实验技术教学指导书籍。

  本书共设实验48项,每项实验内容条理清楚,简明实用,结构完整。按照教学大纲的要求,既介绍了免疫学中的一些经典、传统的实验内容,又增添了目前能开展的先进实验技术(如糖免疫技术,各种免疫细胞纯化技术,肠道、肺部免疫细胞获取,流式细胞仪的多种检测方法应用等)。每项实验包括实验原理、应用、材料、方法、结果、注意事项及思考题等。各项实验绝大部分配有图解,使得实验原理、内容,实验步骤通俗易懂,图文并茂。本书配备了大量编者自己设计的新的图片,使得内容清晰易懂。书后附常用试剂的配方等便于查阅。

  由于本书是国内外第一本医学免疫学双语(中文、英文)实验技术教学指导教材,而且免疫学的发展日新月异,新的发现、新的技术方法和理论层出不穷,因此要编写一本完善的最新免疫学双语教学实验技术指导教材是不容易的。本书的编者在繁忙的工作之余,花了一年的时间与精力,编写了这本双语教材。本书的出版将对免疫学教学的发展起积极的推动作用。

章晓联

2018年8月,武汉

Preface

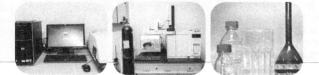

Current Protocols in Immunology A Laboratory Technology in Chinese and English Bilinguals is the latest technical guidance for immunological experiments textbook in Chinese and English and reference for the college students and postgraduates as well as teachers. In order to adapt to the need of integrating Chinese teaching with international teaching, and to popularize bilingual teaching in colleges and universities in China, on the basis of summing up years of experimental teaching experiences, the editor-in-chief organized editors who had studied abroad, are good at English and have abundant teaching experiences in medical immunology to compile this latest bilingual experimental technical guidance of immunology for teaching. Compared with similar books published at home and abroad, this book is characterized by its unique content and English and Chinese expressions, which completely meets the needs of bilingual teaching. This is the urgently needed textbook and reference book for the students and teachers of colleges and universities. It is also the first officially published bilingual (Chinese and English) experimental technology guidance for teaching of medical immunology in China.

There are totally 48 experiments in this textbook. Each experiment is clear, concise and practical, and the structure is complete. And each experiment technique is equipped with a diagrammatic presentation and /or table. According to the requirements of the syllabus, it introduces both classic and traditional experimental contents in medical immunology, as well as practicable advanced experimental techniques (such as glycoimmunology technology, immune cells and intestinal and pulmonary immune cells purification technologies, and techniques for flow cytometry). The book is full of excellent diagrammatic presentation and tables. It is equipped with a large number of new images designed by the editors to make the content easy to be understood. The recipes of commonly used reagents are available at the end of book for reference.

As our knowledge this is the first textbook with experimental technical guide material for bilingual (Chinese and English) medical immunology at home and abroad. The immunological techniques are developed quickly and changed with each passing day. Therefore, it is difficult to compile a perfect latest bilingual technical guidance for immunological experiments textbook. The editors spent one year writing this bilingual textbook which may contain some inadequacies. We hope this book will benefit college students and teachers and will play an important role in promoting the progress of immunology teaching.

Zhang Xiaolian
August 2018, Wuhan

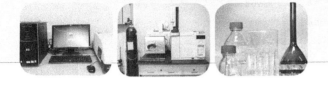

目　录

第一篇　体外抗原抗体反应

1.1　传统的抗原抗体反应 …………………………………………………… 3

　1.1.1　凝集反应 ……………………………………………………………… 4

　　实验一　直接凝集反应——玻片凝集反应鉴定 ABO 血型 ……………… 4

　　实验二　间接凝集反应——测定类风湿因子的乳胶凝集试验 ………… 10

　　实验三　间接凝集抑制反应——测定 HCG 的间接乳胶凝集抑制试验（妊娠
　　　　　　试验） ………………………………………………………………… 14

　1.1.2　沉淀反应 ……………………………………………………………… 18

　　实验四　对流免疫电泳 ……………………………………………………… 18

　　实验五　免疫电泳 …………………………………………………………… 23

　1.1.3　补体参与的抗原抗体反应 ………………………………………… 27

　　实验六　补体凝集素途径测定 …………………………………………… 27

　　实验七　补体溶血空斑试验 ……………………………………………… 32

1.2　功能性细胞因子和免疫球蛋白的检测 …………………………… 39

　　实验八　人血清过敏反应特异性 IgE（SIgE）检测 …………………… 40

1.3　HLA 分型技术 ………………………………………………………… 45

　　实验九　PCR - SSP HLA 分型技术——检测 HLA - B27 基因 ………… 46

第二篇　免疫细胞分离

2.1　免疫细胞的分离和纯化 …………………………………………… 55

　　实验十　外周血单个核细胞分离 ………………………………………… 56

实验十一　小鼠骨髓来源巨噬细胞制备 ················ 60

实验十二　小鼠腹腔巨噬细胞的分离 ················ 64

实验十三　树突状细胞的制备 ················ 69

实验十四　自然杀伤细胞分离 ················ 73

实验十五　磁珠分选小鼠脾脏 T 细胞 ················ 82

实验十六　尼龙棉法分离小鼠 B 细胞 ················ 89

实验十七　磁珠分选 B 细胞 ················ 94

实验十八　小鼠肺泡巨噬细胞的分离和纯化 ················ 98

实验十九　小鼠肠道免疫细胞获取 ················ 103

第三篇　免疫细胞功能检测

实验二十　小鼠脾脏 NK 细胞活性检测 ················ 115

实验二十一　豚鼠 T 细胞 E 玫瑰花环试验 ················ 121

实验二十二　SAP 酶标法测定 T 细胞亚群 ················ 125

实验二十三　单向混合淋巴细胞反应 ················ 130

实验二十四　细胞毒性 T 细胞活性测定 ················ 135

第四篇　抗 体 制 备

实验二十五　多克隆抗体的制备 ················ 143

实验二十六　多克隆抗体的纯化 ················ 147

实验二十七　单克隆抗体制备 ················ 153

实验二十八　单链抗体(scFv)的构建 ················ 162

第五篇　常用的免疫相关疾病动物模型

实验二十九　豚鼠的过敏性休克反应模型 ················ 175

实验三十　Ⅰ型超敏反应小鼠模型——被动皮肤过敏反应 ················ 181

实验三十一　Ⅱ型超敏反应豚鼠模型——Forssman 皮肤血管炎反应 ················ 186

实验三十二　Ⅲ型超敏反应动物模型——Arthus 反应 ················ 190

实验三十三　Ⅳ型超敏反应小鼠模型——二硝基氟苯诱导的迟发型变态反应 ····· 194

实验三十四　小鼠实验性自身免疫性脑脊髓炎的诱导 ················ 198

第六篇　免疫学标记技术

实验三十五　酶联免疫吸附试验 ················ 207

实验三十六　间接免疫荧光法 ·· 212

实验三十七　免疫胶体金技术——测定 HBsAg 的试纸条双抗体夹心法 ········· 216

实验三十八　化学发光免疫标记技术检测乳腺癌患者 HER - 2 胞外结构域
（ECD） ··· 221

实验三十九　生物发光技术 ·· 229

第七篇　细胞凋亡的检测技术和流式细胞术

实验四十　　细胞凋亡的 DNA 琼脂糖凝胶电泳分析 ··································· 237

实验四十一　流式细胞仪检测细胞凋亡——Annexin V /PI 双染色法 ··········· 243

实验四十二　流式细胞术检测小鼠 T 淋巴细胞亚群（CD4$^+$/CD8$^+$T 细胞）
·· 248

实验四十三　流式细胞术检测 CD4$^+$T 细胞上 CXCR4 的表达 ··············· 257

实验四十四　流式细胞仪检测巨噬细胞胞内细胞因子 ······························ 262

第八篇　糖免疫技术

实验四十五　IgG 糖链检测 ·· 271

实验四十六　免疫球蛋白 A1 糖链的检测 ··· 275

实验四十七　细胞表面 N-糖蛋白的代谢标记及检测 ································· 280

实验四十八　胞内 O - GlcNAc 糖蛋白的标记及检测 ································ 284

主要参考文献 ··· 289

附录 ·· 293

　　附录一　常用试剂和培养液 ·· 294

　　附录二　实验常用小鼠的品系及模型 ··· 307

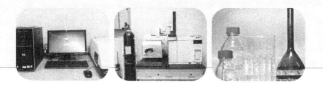

Contents

Chapter One Antigen and Antibody Reaction *in vitro*

1.1 Classical Antigen and Antibody Reaction *in vitro* 3

    1.1.1 Agglutination Reaction 7

    Exp.1 Direct Agglutination Reaction — Slide Agglutination Test for Blood Type Detection 7

    Exp.2 Indirect Agglutination Reaction — Latex Agglutination Test for Detection of RF 12

    Exp.3 Indirect Agglutination Inhibition Reactions — Indirect Latex Agglutination Inhibition Test for the HCG Pregnancy Test 16

    1.1.2 Precipitation Reaction 20

    Exp.4 Countercurrent Electrophoresis 20

    Exp.5 Immunoelectrophoresis 25

    1.1.3 Antigen and Antibody Reaction Involved by Complement 29

    Exp.6 Assay of Complement Lectin Pathway 29

    Exp.7 Hemolytic Plaque Assay 35

1.2 Assay of Functional Cytokine and Immunoglobin 39

    Exp.8 Human Serum Specific IgE (SIgE) Assay for Anaphylaxis 42

1.3 HLA Typing Techniques 45

    Exp.9 HLA Typing for *B27* with PCR − SSP 49

Chapter Two Isolation of Immune Cells

2.1 Separation and Purification of Immune Cells 55

    Exp.10 Separation of Mononuclear Cells from Whole Peripheral Blood 58

Exp.11　Preparation of Mouse Bone Marrow-Derived Macrophages ················ 62

Exp.12　Isolation of Mouse Peritoneal Macrophages ····························· 66

Exp.13　Generation Isolation of Dendritic Cells ································· 71

Exp.14　Isolation of Natural Killer Cells ······································· 77

Exp.15　Isolation of T Cell from Mouse Spleen Using Magnetic Beads ·········· 85

Exp.16　Isolation and Purification of B Cells by Nylon Wool ···················· 91

Exp.17　Isolation and Purification of B Cells by MACS ························· 96

Exp.18　Isolation and Purification of Murine Alveolar Macrophages ············· 100

Exp.19　Isolation of Immune Cells from the Mouse Intestinal Immune System

··· 107

Chapter Three　Assay for the Functions of Immune Cells

Exp.20　Mouse Spleen NK Cells Activity Assay ······························· 118

Exp.21　Erythrocyte Rosette Forming Cell Test (ERFC) for Guinea Pig T
Cells ··· 123

Exp.22　Detection of T Lymphocyte Subgroups in Peripheral Blood by the
SAP ··· 127

Exp.23　One-way Mixed Lymphocyte Reaction ······························· 132

Exp.24　Measurement of CTL Activity ··· 137

Chapter Four　Preparation of Antibody

Exp.25　Preparation of Polyclonal Antibody ·································· 145

Exp.26　Purification of Polyclonal Antibody ·································· 150

Exp.27　Preparation of Monoclonal Antibody ································· 157

Exp.28　Generation of scFv ··· 167

Chapter Five　Animal Models of Immuno-related Diseases

Exp.29　Model of Anaphylaxis Shock in Guinea Pig ························· 178

Exp.30　Murine Model of Type Ⅰ Hypersensitivity Reaction — Passive Cutaneous
Anaphylaxis Model ··· 183

Exp.31　Guinea Pig Type Ⅱ Hypersensitivity Reaction — Forssman Cutaneous
Vasculitis Response ··· 188

Exp.32　Rabbit Type Ⅲ Hypersensitivity Reaction — Arthus Reaction ·········· 192

Exp.33　Mouse Type Ⅳ Hypersensitivity Reaction — Dinitrofluorobenzene-induced Delayed Type Hypersensitivity ·· 196

Exp.34　Induction of Mouse Experimental Autoimmune Encephalomyelitis ······ 201

Chapter Six　Immunolabeling Technique

Exp.35　Enzyme-Linked Immunosorbent Assay（ELISA）··························· 209

Exp.36　Indirect Immunofluorescence Assay ······································· 214

Exp.37　HBsAg Test Trip by Double Antigen Sandwich Immune Colloidal
　　　　Gold Strip Technique ·· 218

Exp.38　Detection of HER-2 Extracellular Domain of Breast Cancer Patients
　　　　by Chemiluminescence Immunoassay ····································· 225

Exp.39　Bioluminescence Assay ·· 232

Chapter Seven　Flow Cytometry and Cell Apoptosis Detection Technique

Exp.40　Thymocytes Apoptosis Assay by Agarose Gel Electrophoresis ··········· 240

Exp.41　Cell Apoptosis Test by Flow Cytometry — Annexin V/PI Dual Staining
　　　　Method ·· 245

Exp.42　Mouse T Lymphocyte Subsets Analysis by Flow Cytometry（CD4$^+$/
　　　　CD8$^+$ T Lymphocytes）·· 252

Exp.43　Flow Cytometry Assay for CXCR4 Expression on CD4$^+$ T Cell ········· 259

Exp.44　Flow Cytometer Analysis for Intracellular Cytokine of Macrophage ······ 265

Chapter Eight　Glycoimmunology Technique

Exp.45　Assay of IgG Sugar Chain ·· 273

Exp.46　Assay of IgA1 Sugar Chain ··· 277

Exp.47　Metabolic Labelling and Detection of N-glycoprotein on Cell Surface ······ 282

Exp.48　Metabolic Labelling and Detection of Intracellular O-GlcNAc
　　　　glycoprotein ·· 286

References ··· 289

Appendices ··· 293

Appendice 1　Commonly Used Reagents and Media ································ 300

Appendice 2　Strains and Models of Mice Commonly Used in Experiments ······ 309

第一篇
Chapter One

体外抗原抗体反应
Antigen and Antibody Reaction *in vitro*

1.1

传统的抗原抗体反应
Classical Antigen and Antibody Reaction *in vitro*

1.1.1

凝 集 反 应

实验一 直接凝集反应——玻片凝集
反应鉴定 ABO 血型

【原理】

凝集反应是颗粒性抗原(如完整的细菌、细胞)与相应抗体,在适当浓度的电解质存在下,经过一定时间,出现肉眼可见的凝集块(图1-1)。

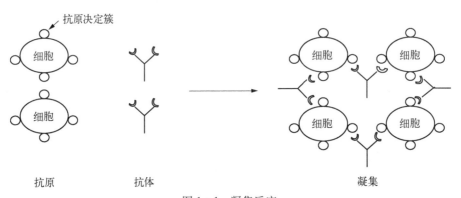

图1-1　凝集反应

玻片凝集试验是在玻片上进行的直接凝集反应。玻片凝集反应是将抗体直接与颗粒性抗原物质(如细菌、红细胞等)混合,在有适当电解质存在的条件下,如两者对应便发生特异性结合而形成肉眼可见的凝集物,即为阳性;如两者不对应便无凝集物出现,即为阴性。

【应用】

玻片凝集反应属定性试验,主要用于细菌的鉴定、分型和人 ABO 血型的鉴定等。本实验是检测人类红细胞表面 A、B 抗原,确定 ABO 血型。

【材料】

1. 抗体:抗 A 和抗 B 标准血清各 1 支
2. 盛有 1 mL 生理盐水(0.9% NaCl)的试管 1 支
3. 消毒针头 1 枚、玻片 1 块、毛细吸管 2 支、75%酒精棉球、灭菌干棉球和 0.5% 84 消毒液

【方法】

1.75%酒精棉球消毒检测者的耳垂或手指尖端,以采血针刺破皮肤,稍加挤压,使血液流出,用毛细吸管取 1~2 滴血液加入含生理盐水的试管内,摇匀,使之成为血细胞悬液。

2. 取一洁净玻片,划分为两格,并标明为"1""2",分别加一滴"抗 A""抗 B"标准血清。

3. 用毛细血管吸取血细胞悬液,在玻片"1"和"2"格各加一滴血细胞悬液。

4. 前后左右不停摇动玻片,使其充分混匀,5 min 后观察有无凝集发生。如肉眼观察难以判断是否有凝集,可在显微镜下用低倍镜观察予以确认。

【结果】

出现凝集颗粒,其周围混合悬液由混浊变为澄清透明者为阳性;如仍呈均匀混浊状者则为阴性(图 1-2)。记录结果,根据表 1-1 判断血型。最后将所用玻片放入置有 84 消毒液的玻片缸中。

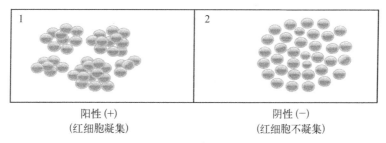

阳性(+)　　　　　　　　　　　　　阴性(-)
(红细胞凝集)　　　　　　　　　　　(红细胞不凝集)

图 1-2　玻片凝集

表 1-1　血型鉴定表

抗 A 标准血清	抗 B 标准血清	血型
-	-	O
+	-	A
-	+	B
+	+	AB

【注意事项】

1. 采血时要严格执行无菌操作。

2. 将含有血液的玻片放置在含有 0.5% 84 消毒液的消毒缸中。

3. 滴加抗体和血液后要充分混匀。

4. 凝集反应出现凝集所需抗体量比沉淀反应所需抗体量少得多。

【思考题】

1. 抗原与抗体反应的特点是什么？影响它们结合的因素是什么？

2. 为什么玻片凝集实验后,玻片必须放入 84 消毒液中？

3. 血型鉴定有什么作用？

(李平飞   章晓联)

Agglutination Reaction

Exp. 1   Direct Agglutination Reaction — Slide Agglutination
Test for Blood Type Detection

【Principle】

Agglutination reaction is the interaction of insoluble particle antigens (e. g. intact bacteria and cells) with specific antibodies to these antigens. In the presence of an appropriate concentration of electrolyte, some visible agglutinates appear in a certain period of time.

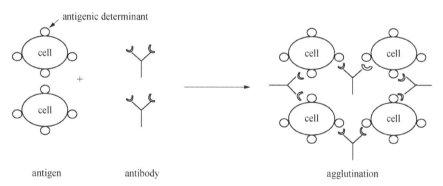

Fig.1 - 1   Agglutination reaction

The slide agglutination test is a direct agglutination reaction performed on a slide. Directly mix antibody with particulate antigenic substance under the certain concentration of electrolyte. The result is positive when there is visible agglutinate, otherwise it is negative.

【Application】

The slide agglutination reaction is a qualitative test, which is mainly used for the identification and classification of bacteria and the identification of human ABO blood type. This experiment is to detect the A, B antigen on the surface of human red blood cells and identify the ABO blood type.

【Materials】

1. Antibody：anti-A, anti-B
2. One tube containing 1 mL of saline (0.9% NaCl)
3. 1 sterilized needle, 1 slide, 2 capillary tubes, 75% alcohol swab and a sterile dry cotton ball

【Procedures】

1. Sterilize the patient's earlobe or finger with 75% alcohol swab, puncture the skin with a needle, squeeze slightly to enable blood flow, take 1 − 2 drops of blood using a capillary tube and trasfer the blood to a test tube containing normal saline. Mix to make blood cell suspension.

2. Divide the clean slide into two panels and label the panels as "1" and "2". Add one drop of "anti-A" and "anti-B" respectively.

3. Pipette the blood cell suspension using a capillary tube, and add a drop of the blood suspension into each of the "1" and "2" wells of the slide.

4. Shake the slides gently, and mix them thoroughly. After 5 mins, observe for a visible agglutination. If it is hard to observe a visible agglutination, it can be confirmed microsopically under low magnification.

【Results】

The result is positive when there is visible agglutination, otherwise it is negative as shown in Fig. 1 − 2. Record the results, and identify blood type according to Tab.1 − 1. Put the slides into the can containing 5% 84 disinfectant solution after the experiments.

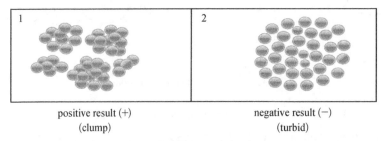

positive result (+)   negative result (−)
(clump)   (turbid)

Fig.1 − 2   Slide agglutination

Tab.1 − 1   Blood type identification table

Anti-A	Anti-B	Blood type
−	−	O
+	−	A
−	+	B
+	+	AB

【Precautions】

1. Strict sterile condition when taking blood samples.

2. Put the slides containing blood into the sterilizing cylinder containing 0.5% 84 disinfectant solution.

3. Mix the suspension thoroughly with antibody solution and blood samples.

4. Much less antibody suffice to produce agglutination than are needed for precipitation.

【Questions】

1. What is the characteristic of the interaction between antigen and antibody? And what are the factors affecting the combination of antigen and antibody?

2. Why do you put the slides into the sterilizing cylinder containing 0.5% 84 disinfectant solution after the experiments?

3. What is the role of blood type identification?

(Li Pingfei   Zhang Xiaolian)

实验二 间接凝集反应——测定类风湿因子的乳胶凝集试验

【原理】

类风湿因子(RF)是类风湿性关节炎患者血清中发现的一组异常的免疫球蛋白,能与人 IgG 的 Fc 部分呈特异性反应。本实验的原理是将人 IgG 结合在载体乳胶颗粒上,当人 IgG 乳胶颗粒与患者血清反应后出现凝集现象,即证明有类风湿因子存在。如将血清连续稀释,能测出血清中类风湿因子的效价。

【应用】

间接凝集试验属定性和半定量试验,用于检测可溶性抗原的特异性抗体。本实验是用已知的人 IgG 致敏乳胶颗粒检测患者血清中的类风湿因子。

【材料】

1. 人 IgG 致敏乳胶颗粒
2. RF 阳性控制血清、阴性控制血清
3. 黑色玻璃板

【方法】

1. 在划格的黑色玻片上,一侧滴加 RF 阳性控制血清,另一侧滴加 RF 阴性控制血清。
2. 将人 IgG 致敏乳胶试剂分别滴加于上述两侧血清,轻轻摇晃玻片,使之混匀。
3. 室温静置 5 min 后,观察结果。

【结果】

阴性对照圈内不出现凝集,试验圈内出现细砂状的乳白色颗粒(图 2-1)。

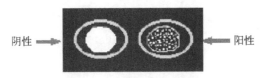

图 2-1 乳胶间接凝集试验

【注意事项】

1. 血清与乳胶试剂要充分混匀。
2. 检测患者的血清时,只有在血清抗体稀释一定比例时才能观察到可见的凝集现象。

【思考题】

1. 乳胶颗粒的存在,会影响阳性血清与人 IgG 的凝集吗?
2. 间接凝集试验可用来检测抗原吗?

（李　群）

Exp. 2　Indirect Agglutination Reaction — Latex Agglutination Test for Detection of RF

【Principle】

Rheumatoid factors (RF) are a group of abnormal immunoglobulins (Igs) in the sera from patients of rheumatoid arthritis. Their antibody activity is directed against antigenic sites in the Fc region of human IgG. The principle of the assay is to coat latex particle with human IgG. If there is agglutination after human IgG latex particle mixed with the test sera, that indicates presence of RF. The patient sera were serially diluted, the approximate titer will correspond to the highest serum dilution exhibiting clearly visible agglutination.

【Application】

Indirect agglutination test is a qualitative and semi-quantitative assay. It is used to detect the specific antibody for the soluble antigen. This assay here is to detect RF in the human sera using known human IgG sensitized latex particle.

【Materials】

1. Human IgG sensitized latex particle
2. RF positive control serum, RF negative control serum
3. Black glass slide

【Procedures】

1. On the black glass slide, place RF positive control on one side and negative control on the other side.

2. Add human IgG sensitized latex particles into the above sera, respectively. Shake the slide gently to mix them well.

3. Leave it for 5 min at room temperature and observe the results.

【Results】

Positive: should exhibit strong agglutination, which will appear as white clumps in a white suspension against a black background.

Negative: exhibit no agglutination, which appears as white homogeneous suspension against a black background (Fig.2 − 1).

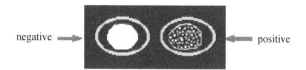

Fig.2 – 1   Latex indirect agglutination test

【Precautions】

1. Sera should be mixed very well with latex reagent.

2. Clear and visible agglutination could only be seen at an appropriate ratio of antibody and antigen (or appropriate dilution of patient sera) when patient sera were measured.

【Questions】

1. Can agglutination appear after positive serum is mixed with human IgG at the presence of latex particle?

2. Can indirect agglutination test be used to detect antigen?

(Li Qun)

实验三 间接凝集抑制反应——测定 HCG 的间接乳胶凝集抑制试验（妊娠试验）

【原理】

间接凝集抑制反应是将待检样品与已知抗体混合并作用一定时间后，再加入相应抗原致敏的载体颗粒，如待检样品中含有相应可溶性抗原，便可先与抗体结合。当再加入抗原致敏颗粒后，因没有相应的抗体，使本应出现的凝集现象被抑制，所以不发生凝集者为阳性结果，表明待检样品中含有相应抗原；发生凝集者为阴性结果，提示待检样品中无相应抗原（图 3-1）。

本实验用间接乳胶凝集抑制试验测定 HCG（妊娠试验）：孕妇尿液中的人绒毛膜促性腺激素（human chorionic gonadotrophin, HCG）与相应的 HCG 抗体充分作用后，再加入 HCG 致敏胶乳，因 HCG 抗体已与尿中 HCG 结合，不再发生凝集反应而呈均匀的乳状液，结果为阳性；如尿液中无 HCG 或含量少，HCG 抗体和 HCG 胶乳发生结合而出现凝集颗粒，结果为阴性。

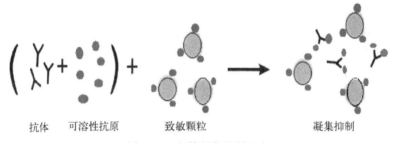

抗体　　可溶性抗原　　致敏颗粒　　　　　　凝集抑制

图 3-1　间接凝集抑制反应

【应用】

间接乳胶凝集抑制试验主要用于检测可溶性抗原 HCG、早期妊娠诊断，也用于辅助诊断宫外孕及不完全流产、滋养层细胞肿瘤、妊娠中毒血症等。

【材料】

1. 聚苯乙烯乳胶抗原（吸附有 HCG），兔抗人 HCG 免疫血清（含 HCG 抗体），生理盐水
2. 待检尿液，孕妇尿液，正常人尿液
3. 黑色玻璃反应板，毛细滴管，牙签、特种铅笔等

【方法】

1. 在黑色玻璃反应板上，用特种铅笔画 3 个直径约 3 cm 的圆圈，并做好标记。圈 1

为待检,圈 2 为阳性对照,圈 3 为阴性对照。

2. 分别滴加待检尿液、孕妇尿液、正常人尿液(或生理盐水)各一滴于圈 1、圈 2 和圈 3 内,然后在三个圈内各滴加免疫血清(HCG 抗体)一滴,分别用牙签混匀,在桌面上连续缓缓摇动 1~2 min。

3. 在三个圈内各滴加胶乳抗原一滴,混匀,再连续摇动 2~5 min,观察结果(图 3-2)。

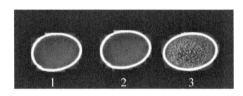

图 3-2 间接乳胶凝集抑制试验(妊娠试验)示意图

【结果】

圈 2(孕妇尿液)含高水平 HCG,HCG 与抗体结合,因此 HCG 包被的乳胶颗粒不发生凝集,为均匀乳胶状无凝集颗粒。圈 3(生理盐水)不含 HCG,抗体与 HCG 包被的颗粒结合,出现明显的均匀一致的细小凝集颗粒。圈 1(待检尿液)如出现明显的均匀一致的凝集颗粒,为阴性结果,说明待检尿液中没有 HCG,即为非妊娠尿;如无凝集颗粒仍呈均匀乳胶状,则为阳性结果,说明待检尿液中有 HCG,即为妊娠尿。肉眼观察不明显时,可借助显微镜观察结果。

【注意事项】

1. 试剂应存放于 2~8℃冰箱中,不能冰冻,否则胶乳上的 HCG 抗原易脱落。
2. 吸取不同样品的毛细滴管和搅拌不同样品的牙签不能混用。
3. 黑色玻璃反应板应平放,圈内加样不宜过多,防止各圈内液体溢流相混。

【思考题】

检测可溶性抗原的方法有哪些?

(王　瑾)

Exp. 3　Indirect Agglutination Inhibition Reactions — Indirect Latex Agglutination Inhibition Test for the HCG Pregnancy Test

【Principle】

Indirect this experiment reaction is to mix the sample with known antibody and incubate for a while, and then add corresponding antigen-sensitized carrier particles. If the antibody is incubated with antigen prior to mixing with antigen-sensitized carrier particle, agglutination is inhibited; this is because free antibodies are not available for agglutination. In this experiment, the absence of agglutination is diagnostic of antigen, and provides a high sensitive assay for small quantities of antigen(Fig.3 − 1).

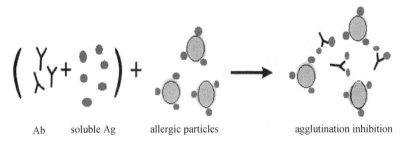

Ab　　　soluble Ag　　allergic particles　　　　　agglutination inhibition

Fig.3 − 1　Indirect agglutination inhibition reaction

This experiment is an indirect latex agglutination inhibition test for the determination of HCG (pregnancy test): A pregnant woman's urine contains HCG (human chorionic gonadotropin) which is secreted by the developing placenta after fertilization. The addition of urine containing HCG, inhibits agglutination of latex particles after added the anti-HCG antibody; and thus the pregnancy is indicated by the absence of agglutination.

【Application】

Indirect latex agglutination inhibition test is mainly used to detect soluble HCG antibody for early pregnancy diagnosis, also used to assist in the diagnosis of ectopic pregnancy and incomplete abortion, trophoblastic tumor, gestational toxemia, etc.

【Materials】

1. HCG-coated latex particles, rabbit anti-human HCG immune serum, normal urine
2. Urine to be tested, urine of pregnant women, normal human urine
3. Black glass slide, capillary dropper, toothpick, special pencil, etc.

【Procedures】

1. Draw three circles of about 3 cm in diameter on a black glass slide and label them with special pencil. circle 1: to be tested; circle 2: positive control; circle 3: negative control.

2. One drop of urinary samples, pregnant urine, and normal human urine (normal saline) is added to the circle 1, circle 2 and circle 3 respectively, and then one drop of rabbit anti-human HCG immune serum is added to each of the three circles and incubate minutes.

3. Add a drop of latex antigen to each of the three circles, mix well, and shake continuously for 2 − 5 minutes to observe the results(Fig.3 − 2).

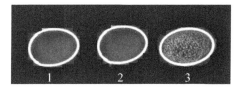

Fig.3 − 2   Indirect latex agglutination inhibition test (pregnancy test)

【Results】

Circle 2(pregnant urine): The level of HCG is high, will bind with the antibodies, and thus no agglutination with the HCG-coated latex particles occurs.

Circle 3(normal saline): The level of HCG is too low, the antibodies will remain to agglutinate the HCG-coated latex particles, and the agglutination occurs.

Circle 1 (urine to be tested): if agglutination occurs, it is a negative result, indicating that there is no HCG in the urine to be tested. If no agglutination occurs, it is a positive result, indicating that there is HCG in the urine to be tested.

【Precautions】

1. Reagents should be stored in a refrigerator at $2 - 8\,^{\circ}\!C$, not frozen, otherwise the HCG antigen on the latex is easy to fall off.

2. Capillary droppers and toothpicks used cannot be mixed.

3. The black glass slide should be laid flat, and do not add too much sample in the circles.

【Question】

What are the methods for detecting soluble antigens?

(Ma Yunfeng   Ji Yanhong)

1.1.2

沉 淀 反 应

实验四　　对流免疫电泳

【原理】

　　对流免疫电泳是双向琼脂扩散与电泳技术的结合。抗原或抗体分子在一定的 pH 溶液中带有电荷,在电场作用下可发生定向移动。将抗原、抗体分别加在 pH 为 8.6 的琼脂中电泳,因各种血清蛋白都带负电荷,泳向阳极。由于电渗作用,液体则流向阴极,二者方向相反。抗体(多为丙种球蛋白)的等电点较高(pI 6~7),故带负电荷少,又因分子量大,所以电泳力小于电渗力,向阴极移动。而抗原的等电点较低(pI 4~5),所带负电荷多,又因其分子量较小,故其电泳力大于电渗力,向正极移动。如抗原、抗体相遇,在比例适当时即形成白色沉淀线。由于电场限制了抗原、抗体分子的自由扩散,因而提高了试验的敏感性(提高 10~20 倍),并缩短了反应时间(与双向琼脂扩散相比)。

【应用】

　　对多种抗原、抗体进行定性及半定量检测。

【材料】

　　1. 抗原:待测人血清,甲胎蛋白阳性血清
　　2. 抗体:甲胎蛋白诊断血清(抗甲胎蛋白抗体)
　　3. 巴比妥缓冲液(0.05 mol/L, pH 8.6)、0.4%巴比妥琼脂、1.5%巴比妥琼脂
　　4. 其他:电泳仪、打孔器、载玻片、毛细吸管、电表等

【方法】

　　1. 制板:取一洁净载玻片,先用 0.4%巴比妥琼脂铺底、烘干,放置水平台面上。再取 4 mL 煮溶的 1.5%巴比妥琼脂,立即浇注在已铺底的玻片上,制成厚薄均匀的琼脂板。
　　2. 打孔:待琼脂凝固后,用打孔器按图 4-1 打孔,孔径 3 mm,孔距 5 mm。
　　3. 加样:用毛细吸管取待检血清(抗原)10 μL 分别加于阴极侧 1、2、3 孔内,甲胎蛋

白阳性血清如肝癌病人阳性血清 10 μL 加于 4 孔内作为对照,阳极侧 5、6、7、8 各孔均加甲胎蛋白诊断血清。加样量以孔满为宜,但不可溢出孔外。

4. 电泳:琼脂板放入电泳槽内,琼脂板两端用滤纸或纱布与缓冲液相接,抗原端接负极电源,抗体端接正极电源。按电场强度 4~6 V/cm 电泳 50 min 左右。

【结果】

电泳完毕,关闭电源,取出琼脂板,在黑色背景下观察,凡抗原抗体孔间出现白色沉淀线者为阳性(+),孔间无白色沉淀线者为阴性(-)。如沉淀线不清晰可将琼脂板置 37℃温箱数小时后再进行观察,也可染色观察(图 4-1)。

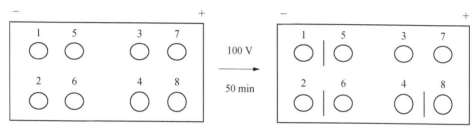

图 4-1　对流免疫电泳

【注意事项】

1. 根据配制琼脂的缓冲液的离子类型和离子强度不同,对流免疫电泳可分为连续电泳和不连续电泳两种。连续电泳槽液与配琼脂的缓冲液相同,不连续电泳槽液离子强度高于配制琼脂的缓冲液离子强度。实验证明不连续电泳具有电泳快、形成沉淀线清晰、电渗失水不明显等优点。

2. 在抗原与抗体孔间出现沉淀线者为阳性。沉淀线形状、位置等差异,与抗原、抗体浓度及分子量有关。

【思考题】

对流免疫电泳中,抗原端为何接负极?

（章晓联）

Precipitation Reaction

Exp. 4   Countercurrent Electrophoresis

【Principle】

Countercurrent electrophoresis is performed in agar gels where the pH is chosen so that the antibody is positively charged and the antigen being tested is negatively charged. By applying a voltage across the gel, the antigen and antibody move towards each other and precipitate. Antibody is usually added at anode (+) side, while the antigen is usually added at cathode (−) side. This is because the antibodies (IgGs) usually carry low negative charge in the electrophoresis buffer with pH 8.6 since the values of their pIs are usually at 6−7 and the molecular weight of the antibodies is high, so the electrophoresis mobility of the antibodies is lower than its electro-osmotic mobility. While antigens usually carry high negative charges in the pH8.6 of electrophoresis buffer since the values of their pIs are usually at 4−5 and the molecular weight of the antigens is low, so the electrophoresis mobility of the antigens is larger than its electro-osmotic mobility.

The sensitivity of countercurrent electrophoresis is increased 10−20 times more than the double immunodiffusion and the time of the experiment is shorter than that of the double immunodiffusion.

【Application】

Countercurrent electrophoresis can be used to identify the antigens or antibodies with quantity.

【Materials】

1. Antigen (Ag): unknown human serum, AFP (alpha fetoprotein) positive human serum

2. Antibody (Ab): AFP diagnostic serum (anti-AFP)

3. Barbital buffer (0. 05 mol/L, pH 8. 6), 0. 4% barbital agar, 1. 5% barbital agar

4. Others: electrophoresis apparatus, slide, puncher, capillary pipette and electro-meter, etc.

【Procedures】

1. Prepare agar plate: 0. 4% barbital agar is poured on the slide as bedding. The slide is dried and again overlaid with 4 mL melted 1. 5% barbital agar.

2. Punch wells: after the agar solidified, wells are bored by puncher according to Fig.4−1 whose bore diameter is 3 mm and bore distance 5 mm.

3. Add samples: add 10 μL antigen (unknown human serum) to the wells "1", "2", "3" at cathode (−) side with micropipette. Add 10 μL antigen AFP positive human serum, e. g. hepatitis positive patient serum, to the well "4" as control well. Add 10 μL AFP diagnostic serum to the wells "5", "6", "7" and "8" at anode (+) side. Don't overload samples outside the wells.

4. Electrophoresis: put the agar plate in the electrophoresis apparatus. Use filter paper or gauze to link the barbital buffer and agar plate. Apply voltage at 4−6 V/cm for 50 min.

【Results】

Switch off the power. Put the agar plate above the black background. White precipitin line observed represents positive result (+). No precipitin line represents negative result (−) (Fig.4−1). If the precipitation is not clear, the slide can be placed in a 37℃ incubator for several hours before observation. It can also be observed by staining.

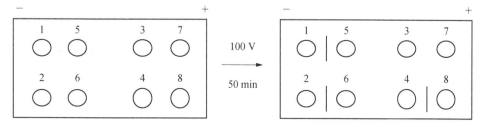

Fig.4−1　Countercurrent electrophoresis

【Precautions】

1. Countercurrent electrophoresis can be divided into two types. One is a continuous electrophoresis, while the other is an incontinuous electrophoresis, based on the ions' characteristics. The electrophoresis buffers are the same as the agar buffers in the continuous electrophoresis, while the electrophoresis buffers' ion strength is higher than that of agar buffers in the incontinuous electrophoresis. It is demonstrated that it is faster when you run the electrophoresis and it can form clear precipitate line in the incontinuous electrophoresis

system.

2. When you observe precipitin line between the wells of antigen and antibody, it represents positive result (+). The shape and position of the precipitin line are related with the concentration and molecular weight of the antigen and the antibody.

【Question】

Why put antigen on the cathode side?

(Zhang Xiaolian)

实验五 免疫电泳

【原理】

免疫电泳是电泳和双向免疫扩散相结合的一种抗原分析方法。先将待测抗原加入琼脂板小孔中进行电泳,因电泳速度不同可将待测抗原中的不同组分分开,然后再与横槽中已知抗体进行双向扩散,每一对相应的抗原、抗体结合形成一条沉淀弧(图5-1)。根据弧的数目、形状和位置,可分析样品中的抗原成分及性质。

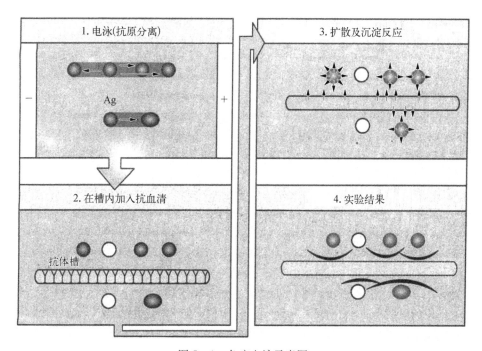

图5-1 免疫电泳示意图

【应用】

用于某种组分分析及纯度的鉴定。下面以检测人血清为例介绍免疫电泳。

【材料】

1. 抗原:待测人血清、标准人血清
2. 抗体:抗人血清抗体
3. 其他:巴比妥缓冲液(离子强度 0.05 mol/L,pH 8.6)、0.4%巴比妥琼脂、1.5%巴比妥琼脂、载玻片、打孔器、微量加样器、电泳仪等

【方法】

1. 制板：取一洁净载玻片，用0.4%巴比妥琼脂铺底，待干。于玻片中央置一小玻棒，取1.5%巴比妥琼脂3.5 mL浇板，待凝固后打孔。
2. 加抗原：用微量加样器每孔加入抗原10 μL。
3. 电泳：抗原孔放负极端，按电压4~6 V/cm电泳1~1.5 h。
4. 加抗体：开槽后，加入抗体充满小槽。
5. 扩散：将琼脂板置湿盒中，37℃扩散24~72 h，至沉淀弧清晰为止。

【结果】

扩散完后，记录沉淀弧的数目、位置和形状，并与标准品比较。

【注意事项】

1. 抗原、抗体的比例：如同其他沉淀反应一样，要预测最佳抗原、抗体量。
2. 抗血清的抗体谱：一只动物的抗血清往往缺乏某些抗体，若将几只动物的抗血清混合使用，则效果更好。
3. 电泳条件：如缓冲液、琼脂、电流等皆可直接影响沉淀弧的分辨率。

【思考题】

先天性丙种球蛋白缺乏症患者的免疫电泳图形有什么特点？

（刘　春）

Exp. 5　Immunoelectrophoresis

【Principle】

The technique of immunoelectrophoresis combines electrophoresis with double immunodiffusion. An antigen mixture is first analyzed by electrophoresis to separate its components according to the electric charge. Troughs are then cut into the agar parallel to the direction of the troughs. Antibody and antigen then diffuse toward each other and produce precipitin arc where they meet in appropriate proportions (Fig.5 − 1).

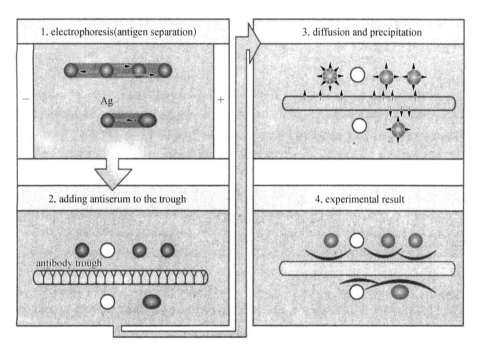

Fig.5 − 1　Immunoelectrophoresis

【Application】

The technique of immunoelectrophoresis is used to detect the presence or absence or purity of proteins in the serum. We introduce the technique by way of detecting the proteins of human serum.

【Materials】

1. Antigen: patient serum, standard human serum
2. Antibody: goat anti-human serum

3. Others: 0.05 mol/L barbital buffer (pH8.6), 0.4% and 1.5% barbital agar, and slide, puncher, micropipette and electrophoresis apparatus

【Procedures】

1. Prepare agar plate: 0.4% barbital agar is poured on the slide as bedding. Once the slide is dried, put the glass stick in the middle of the slide, and then add another layer of 1.5% barbital agar. After the agar is solidified, wells are punched by the puncher.

2. Add antigen: 10 μL antigen is added to every well with micropipette.

3. Electrophoresis: antigen in cathode well is analysed by electrophoresis at voltage 4 to 6 V/cm for 60 – 90 min.

4. Add antibody: following electrophoresis, troughs are cut into the agar parallel to the direction of the electric filled, and are filled with antibody.

5. Diffuse: the agar plate in a humidified box is diffused for 24 to 72 h at 37℃ and waits till precipitin arcs become distinct.

【Results】

After diffusion, the number, position and shape of precipitin arcs of patient serum are recorded and compared with standard human serum.

【Precautions】

Many factors affect the position, shape and distinctness of precipitin arcs: ① the proportion of antigen and antibody; ② the antibody broadness of antiserum; ③ Electrophoresis condition: such as the barbital buffer, agar and current.

【Question】

What is the characteristic of the immunoelectrophoretic pattern of serum from patients with congenital gamma-globulin deficiency?

(Liu Chun)

1.1.3

补体参与的抗原抗体反应

实验六　　补体凝集素途径测定

【原理】

补体凝集素途径和经典途径中都有 C4 补体的裂解、活化并产生 C4c 片段,高盐环境可抑制补体经典途径。由于 C4 在补体旁路途径中不存在,所以在高盐环境中 C4c 在细胞表面的沉积可以代表补体凝集素途径的活性(图 6-1)。

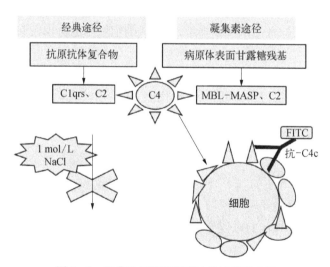

图 6-1　经典途径和凝集素途径过程示意图

【应用】

检测补体凝集素途径的功能,判断补体凝集素系统的激活。

【材料】

1. 鼠伤寒沙门菌 C5

2. 血清稀释缓冲液：Tris-HCl 20 mmol/L，NaCl 1 mol/L，CaCl$_2$ 10 mmol/L，0.05%（V/V）TritonX－100，0.1%（m/V）BSA

3. C4 蛋白溶解液：巴比妥 4 mmol/L，NaCl 145 mmol/L，CaCl$_2$ 2 mmol/L，MgCl$_2$ 1 mmol/L

4. MBL/Ficolin 20 μg/mL，C4 蛋白，GST 蛋白

5. FITC 标记的抗 C4c

6. GlcNAc（N-乙酰葡糖胺）琼脂糖和甘露糖琼脂糖

7. 4℃离心机、4℃层析柜、37℃孵育箱和流式细胞仪

【方法】

1. 血清制备：取新鲜的健康人血清，用稀释缓冲液稀释（50%稀释）后，加入 GlcNAc 琼脂糖和甘露糖琼脂糖，室温下振荡反应 30 min，4℃、7 250 r/min 离心 5 min，取上清。

2. 取 10^8 个鼠伤寒沙门菌 C5，PBS 洗两遍，弃上清，每管加入以上处理好的血清 100 μL，同时加入 20 μg/mL MBL/Ficolin 100 μL，或等量的 GST 蛋白作为对照组，4℃孵育过夜。

3. 13 000 r/min，离心 4 min，并用 PBS 洗 1 次后，每管加入 1 mg/mL 的 C4 补体蛋白（用 C4 蛋白溶解液稀释）100 μL，37℃孵育 1.5 h，并用 PBS 洗 1 次。

4. 每管加入按 1∶100 稀释的 FITC 标记的抗 C4c 补体的荧光抗体 100 μL，37℃作用 30 min，PBS 洗 2 次后用 100 μL PBS 重悬，用流式细胞仪测定沉积在细菌上的 C4c。

【结果】

与 GST 组比较，实验组的 C4c 阳性率代表 MBL/Ficolin 激活补体凝集素途径的能力。

【注意事项】

1. 鼠伤寒沙门菌 C5 中的"C5"不是补体，而是细菌名称。

2. 加入各种试剂之后要轻轻混匀。

3. 孵育染流式荧光抗体的时候要避光。

【思考题】

1. 该实验除了检测凝集素对补体的激活作用外，还可以检测血清的补体活性吗？

2. 加入的健康人血清有什么作用？

（吴　剑　章晓联）

1.1.3

Antigen and Antibody Reaction Involved by Complement

Exp. 6　Assay of Complement Lectin Pathway

【Principle】

Cleavage, activation of complement C4 and production of C4c fragment are occurred in both classical pathway and lectin pathway of complement activation. The classical pathway of complement is inhibited in a high concentration of salt. In high salt environment, deposition of C4c on the cell surface indicates the activity of complement lectin pathway, because C4 does not participate in the alternative complement pathway(Fig.6−1).

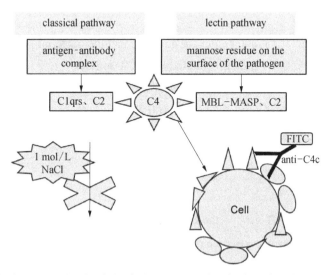

Fig.6−1　The block of classical pathway and activation of lectin pathway

【Application】

Examine the function of the complement lectin pathway and determine the activation of the complement lectin pathway.

【Materials】

1. *Salmonella typhimurium* C5

2. Serum dilution buffer: Tris-HCl 20 mmol/L, NaCl 1 mol/L, CaCl$_2$ 10 mmol/L, 0.05% (*V/V*) Triton X-100, 0.1% (*m/V*) BSA

3. C4 protein solution: barbital 4 mmol/L, NaCl 145 mmol/L, CaCl$_2$ 2 mmol/L, MgCl$_2$ 1 mmol/L

4. 20 μg/mL MBL/Ficolin, C4 protein, GST protein

5. FITC-anti C4c

6. GlcNAc-agarose and mannose-agarose

7. 4℃ centrifuge, 4℃ chromatography cabinet, 37℃ incubator and flow cytometer

【Procedures】

1. Serum preparation: dilute fresh healthy human serum with dilution buffer (50% dilution). Add GlcNAc (N-acetylglucosamine)-agarose and mannose agarose into the serum. Shake at room temperature for 30 min and centrifuge the serum at 4℃ 7 250 r/min for 5 min. Collect the supernatant.

2. Wash 10^8 *Salmonella typhimurium* C5 with PBS twice. Discard the supernatant, and add 100 μL of the above serum (STEP 1) to each tube. Add 20 μg/mL lectin MBL/Ficolin 100 μL or the same amount of GST protein (control) into the tube, and incubate at 4℃ overnight.

3. After centrifuge at 13,000 r/min for 4 min, wash the bacterial pellets once with PBS. Add 100 μL of 1 mg/mL C4 protein (diluted with C4 solution) to each tube, and incubate the mixture at 37℃ for 1.5 h. Then wash bacterial pellets with PBS.

4. Add 100 μL of FITC-anti C4c (1 : 100 dilution) to each tube, and incubate the tubes at 37℃ for 30 min. Wash the bacterial pellets with PBS twice, suspend the cells in 100 μL PBS, and measure the C4c deposited on bacteria by flow cytometer.

【Results】

Compared with the GST group, the C4c positive rate of the experimental group indicates the ability of the complement lectin activation by MBL/Ficolin.

【Precautions】

1. The "C5" in *Salmonella typhimurium* C5 is not a complement but a bacterial name.

2. Mix gently after adding reagents.

3. Fluorescent antibody staining should be incubated in the dark.

【Questions】

1. In addition to assay the activation of complement by lectin, can this experiment be used to detect the activity of serum complement?

2. What is the function of healthy human serum?

(Wu Jian   Zhang Xiaolian)

实验七　补体溶血空斑试验

【原理】

绵羊红细胞(SRBC)免疫的小鼠脾细胞,与琼脂糖凝胶中的 SRBC 共同孵育,脾细胞中的抗体形成细胞合成并分泌抗 SRBC 的抗体,再加入补体时,在抗体形成细胞周围的结合有抗体的 SRBC 被补体溶解,产生溶血空斑(图 7-1)。

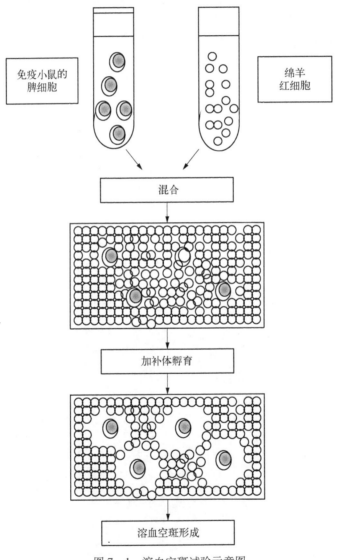

图 7-1　溶血空斑试验示意图

【应用】

此法可用于研究体内抗体产生能力。例如,能研究一些药物对抗体产生的调节效应。

【材料】

1. 绵羊红细胞(SRBC,保存于 Alsever's 液)
2. 小鼠(18~20 g)
3. 豚鼠血清(作为补体)
4. 琼脂糖(1% m/V,用蒸馏水配制)
5. 0.14 mol/L 氯化钠溶液
6. Hank's 液
7. Earle's 液
8. Alsever's 红细胞保存液
9. 2 倍浓缩的 RPMI-1640 培养液
10. 不锈钢网(200 目)
11. 湿盒
12. 注射器内芯、培养皿、试管、吸管、载玻片、水浴箱等

【方法】

1. 实验前 5 天以 1 mL 5% SRBC 经腹腔免疫 2 只小鼠。
2. 用 Hank's 液洗涤 SRBC 3 次,1 000 r/min 离心 10 min,配成 10% V/V。
3. 取免疫小鼠脾脏,置培养皿中的 200 目不锈钢网上,用注射器内芯将脾脏轻轻压过钢网,取出钢网,用吸管轻轻吹吸分散细胞。
4. 将脾细胞悬液移至试管,用 Earle's 液洗 1 次,1 000 r/min 离心 10 min。
5. 弃上清,用 Earle's 液重悬脾细胞,配成 1×10^7 细胞/mL 的悬液。
6. 1% 琼脂糖溶化后,加入等量预热的 2 倍浓缩的 RPMI-1640 培养液,立即摇匀,置 45℃ 水浴箱中备用。
7. 小玻璃试管中加入 10%SRBC 0.05 mL,脾细胞悬液 0.1 mL,置 45℃ 水浴中混匀,再用预热的吸管加上述 RPMI-1640 培养液与琼脂糖液的混合液 0.4 mL,仍在水浴中充分混匀。
8. 载玻片置于平台上,迅速将混合物倒于载玻片上,使之铺平。
9. 待凝固后置湿盒内,37℃ 中温育 30 min。
10. 加 1∶10 稀释的豚鼠血清 1 mL,继续温育 2 h。

【结果】

肉眼可见的边缘整齐的圆形透亮区为空斑,显微镜下可见空斑的中央为分泌抗体的细胞。在双目低倍显微镜下计数每张玻片的空斑数,算出每百万个脾细胞中的空斑形成细胞数。

【注意事项】

1. 如果从孵箱中取出载玻片时未见明显溶血空斑出现,可在室温中放置 30 min 后,再看结果。

2. 实验全过程中须保持脾细胞的活性。

3. 含有脾细胞、SRBC、琼脂糖和 RPMI－1640 培养液的混合物须保持在 45℃水浴中,并快速均匀地倾倒在置于平台上的载玻片上。

4. 载玻片须放于湿盒内进行温育,防止干燥。

5. 上述方法只能检测直接空斑(主要为 IgM),检测间接空斑(IgG)需加入抗小鼠 Ig 的抗体,如能得到合适的抗体,间接空斑能检测小鼠的所有 IgG 亚类。

【思考题】

如果出现很少的空斑,其原因是什么?

（田野平）

Exp. 7   Hemolytic Plaque Assay

【Principle】

Splenocytes from the mice immunized by sheep red blood cells (SRBC) are incubated with SRBC in an agarose gel. Antibody-producing cells in the splenocytes synthesize and secrete antibodies against SRBC during the incubation. After the addition of complement, the erythrocytes bound antibodies in the locality of the antibody-producing cells are lysed and the plaques or holes appear in the agarose gel with erythrocyte suspension (Fig.7 − 1).

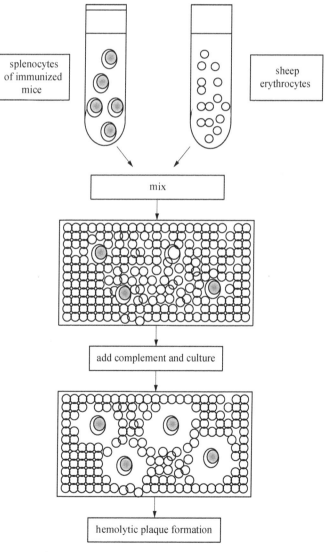

Fig.7 − 1   Sketch map of hemolytic plaque assay

【Application】

The hemolytic plaque assay can be used to evaluate the ability of antibody production in the body. For example, the regulatory effects of some drugs on the antibody production can be investigated by hemolytic plaque assay.

【Materials】

1. Sheep erythrocytes, SRBC, in Alsever's solution
2. Mice, 18 – 20 g
3. Guinea-pig serum, as complement source
4. Agarose, 1% m/V in distilled water
5. 0. 14 mol/L NaCl solution
6. Hank's solution
7. Earle's solution
8. Alsever's solution
9. 2×RPMI – 1640 medium
10. Stainless steel 200 – mesh screen
11. Humidified box
12. Syringe core, culture dishes, test tubes, pipettes, slides, water bath, etc.

【Procedures】

1. Immunize 2 mice with 1 mL of 5% sheep erythrocytes given intraperitoneally 5 days before the experiment.

2. Wash sheep erythrocytes in Hank's saline (three times at 1,000 r/min for 10 min) and dilute to 10% V/V.

3. Remove spleen from immunized mouse and put it on a stainless steel 200-mesh screen in a dish. Add a little Earle's solution into the dish and push the spleen slightly through the screen with the flat top surface of a syringe core. Take out the screen and suck the splenocyte suspension in and out of a pipette to disperse the cells.

4. Transfer the splenocyte suspension into a glass test tube. Wash the splenocytes once with Earle's solution by centrifugation at 1,000 r/min for 10 min.

5. Discard the supernatant and re-suspend packed cells in Earle's solution. Adjust to 1×10^7 cells/mL.

6. Mix 1% melted agarose with equivalent 2×RPMI – 1640 medium in a 45℃ water bath immediately.

7. Add 0. 1 mL splenocyte suspension into a small glass test tube containing 0. 05 mL of 10% SRBC in a 45℃ water bath. Then, add 0. 4 mL above medium-agarose into this test tube containing splenocytes and SRBC by a hot pipette and mix thoroughly in a 45℃ water

bath.

8. Place slides covered by agar underlay on a leveled surface. Pour above mixture out of the small glass test tube and spread on the slide.

9. Allow agarose to harden and incubate the slides in a humidified box at 37℃ for half an hour.

10. Add 1. 0 mL of a 1 ∶ 10 dilution of guinea-pig serum as a source of complement and incubate the slide continuously at 37℃ for 2 h.

【Results】

The formation of circular clear zones in a background of un-lysed SRBC is macroscopic. The antibody-secreting cell located in the center of a plaque can be observed with microscope.

Counting is easier if you use a low-power binocular microscope and draw lines on the bottom of the slide. Calculate the number of plaque-forming cells (PFC) per 10^6 splenocytes.

【Precautions】

1. If the plaques are not clear when the slides are taken out from the incubator, put them in room temperature for about 30 min before counting.

2. Keep the viability of the splenocytes during the whole experiment.

3. Maintain the mixture containing agarose gel, SRBC, splenocytes and medium at 45℃ water bath. Pour the mixture on a slide quickly and evenly.

4. Place the slide in a humidified condition to protect it from dry.

5. Only direct plaques (mainly IgM antibody) are detected by the method described above. To detect IgG plaques it is necessary to use an antiserum against mouse Ig. This method detecting so-called "indirect" plaques can be used to assay all mouse IgG subclasses if the appropriate antisera are available.

【Question】

What are the reasons if few plaques appear?

(Tian Yeping)

功能性细胞因子和免疫球蛋白的检测

Assay of Functional Cytokine and Immunoglobin

实验八　人血清过敏反应特异性 IgE（SIgE）检测

【原理】

采用 ELISA 法,将相应抗原包被在酶标板上,然后加入待测血清和生物素标记的特异性抗 IgE 抗体,洗涤后,加入链霉素标记的 HRP,最后加入底物,产生颜色(图 8-1)。颜色的深浅和血清样品中 IgE 的浓度呈正比。

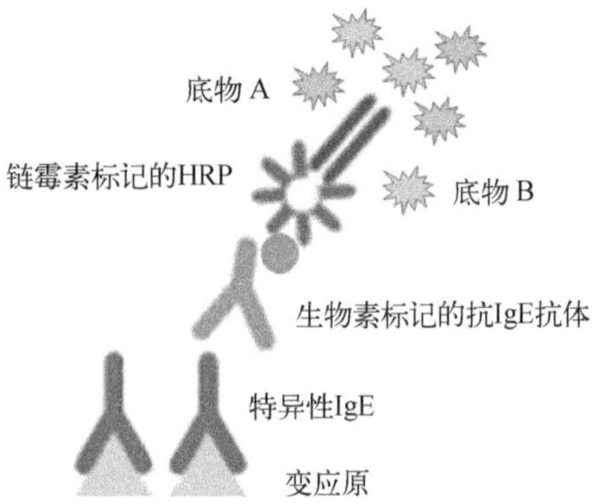

【应用】

诊断过敏反应,确定过敏原。

【材料】

1. 人血清特异性 IgE(SIgE)ELISA 试剂盒
2. 蒸馏水、加样器
3. 振荡器、酶标仪等

图 8-1　检测血清 IgE 示意图

【方法】

1. 待测标本用标本稀释液 1:1 稀释后,取 50 μL 加于反应孔内,其他反应孔加入稀释好后的标准品 50 μL。

2. 立即在每个反应孔中加入 50 μL 生物素标记的抗 IgE 抗体。盖上封口膜,轻轻振荡混匀,37℃温育 1 h。

3. 甩去反应孔内液体,每个反应孔加满洗涤液,振荡 30 s,甩去洗涤液后用吸水纸拍干。重复此操作 3 次。

4. 每个反应孔加入 50 μL 链霉素标记的 HRP,轻轻振荡混匀,37℃温育 30 min。

5. 甩去反应孔内液体,每个反应孔加满洗涤液,振荡 30 s,甩去洗涤液后用吸水纸拍干。重复此操作 3 次。

6. 每个反应孔加入底物 A、底物 B 各 50 μL,轻轻振荡混匀,37℃温育 10 min。避免光照。

7. 取出酶标板,迅速加入 50 μL 终止液,加入终止液后应立即测定结果。

【结果】

1. 仪器值:于波长 450 nm 的酶标仪上读取各反应孔的 OD 值。

2. 以吸光度 OD 值为纵坐标(Y),相应的待测物质标准品浓度为横坐标(X),得到相应曲线,样品的待测物质含量可根据其 OD 值由标准曲线换算出相应的浓度。

【注意事项】

1. 底物 A 易挥发,避免长时间打开盖子。底物 B 对光敏感,避免长时间暴露于光下。避免用手接触,有毒。

2. 实验完成后应立即读取 OD_{450} 值。

【思考题】

血清特异性 IgE（SIgE)检测是否能准确反映患者的致敏状态?

（罗凤玲）

Human Serum Specific IgE （SIgE）
Assay for Anaphylaxis

【**Principle**】

Using ELISA, the corresponding antigen was coated on the ELISA plates, then patient
sera and specific biotin labelled anti-IgE
antibodies were added. After washing,
streptomycin labelled HRP was added,
and substrates were finally added to
produce color (Fig. 8 – 1). The depth of
color is proportional to the IgE
concentration in the serum sample.

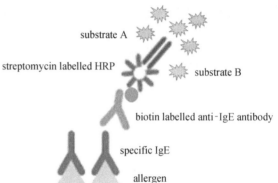

【**Application**】

Diagnose allergic reactions and identify
allergens.

Fig. 8 – 1　Schematic diagram of serum IgE assay

【**Materials**】

1. Human serum specific IgE (SIgE) assay kit
2. Distilled water, pipettes
3. Oscillator, microplate reader, etc.

【**Procedures**】

1. Samples were diluted at 1 ：1, and 50 μL diluted samples were added to the wells.
Other reaction wells are added with diluted standards.

2. 50 μL biotin labelled IgE antibodies were added in each well immediately, cover the
lid and mixed gently and incubate at 37℃ for 1 h.

3. Shake off the liquid in the well, fill each well with washing buffer, oscillate for 30 s,
shake off the washing liquid and dry with absorbent paper. Repeat this three times.

4. 50 μL streptomycin labeled HRP were added in each well, mix gently, incubate at
37℃ for 1 h. Avoid light.

5. Shake off the liquid in the well, fill each well with washing buffer, oscillate for 30 s,
shake off the washing liquid and dry with absorbent paper. Repeat this three times.

6. 50 μL substrate A and B were added in each well. Mix gently, incubate at 37℃ for
1 h. Avoid light.

7. Take out the plate, quickly add 50 μL terminated liquid, and determine the results immediately.

[Results]

1. OD value of each well was measured with microplate reader at 450 nm wavelength.

2. Taking the absorbance OD value as the vertical coordinate (Y) and the concentration of the standard substance as the horizontal coordinate (X), and the corresponding curve is made. The content of the substance to be measured can be converted from the standard curve according to its OD value.

[Precautions]

1. Substrate A is volatile. Avoiding opening the lid for a long time. Substrate B is sensitive to light. Avoiding prolonged exposure to light. Avoid contact because they are toxic.

2. The OD_{450} value should be read immediately.

[Question]

Whether serum specific IgE (SIgE) assay can accurately reflect the patient's sensitization state?

(Luo Fengling)

1.3

HLA 分型技术
HLA Typing Techniques

实验九   PCR - SSP HLA 分型技术——检测 *HLA - B27* 基因

【原理】

人类 *HLA* 基因具有丰富的多态性。在一个随机人群中每一个基因座位上都有很多等位基因,而每一个等位基因又有其各自独特的 DNA 序列。

根据 *HLA* 等位基因碱基序列设计并合成与之互补寡核苷酸作为 PCR 引物即序列特异性引物(SSP),该引物能和 DNA 样本中的互补序列特异性地结合并通过 PCR 进行扩增,PCR 扩增产物的出现提示样品中待测的 *HLA* 等位基因的存在。图 9 - 1 ~ 图 9 - 4 是 PCR - SSP HLA 分型技术检测 *HLA - B27* 基因的操作流程。

取全血
↓
裂解 RBC,收集有核细胞(白细胞)
↓
消化蛋白酶 K,释放 DNA 出细胞核
↓
DNA 溶解于液相,可用做 DNA 模板
↓
用 *HLA - B27* 的 SSP 进行 PCR 扩增
↓
凝胶电泳检测 PCR 产物
↓
如果凝胶中有 PCR 产物,提示样品为 *HLA - B27*(+)
如果凝胶中无 PCR 产物,提示样品为 *HLA - B27*(-)

图 9 - 1   HLA 分型的流程图

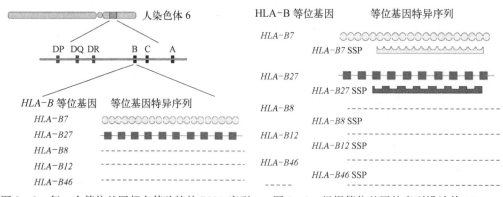

图 9 - 2   每一个等位基因都有其独特的 DNA 序列   图 9 - 3   根据等位基因的序列设计其 SSP

【应用】

1. 用于同种异型移植的组织配型。

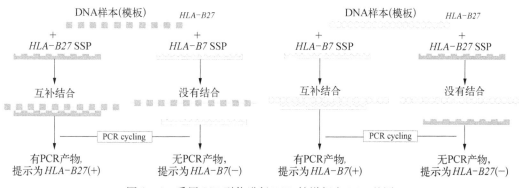

图 9－4　采用 SSP 引物进行 PCR 扩增相应 HLA 基因

2. 用于 HLA 相关疾病的研究。

3. 用于法医学和人类学的研究。

【材料】

1. EDTA 抗凝的全血 0.2 mL, HLA－B27 阳性对照

2. RBC 裂解缓冲液

3. WBC 裂解缓冲液

4. PCR 混合液

5. 加样缓冲液(甲酚红,终浓度为 0.001%, m/V)

6. 离心管、试管吸管、离心机、PCR 仪等

【方法】

1. DNA 提取:从样品的白细胞中提取 DNA,用作 PCR 扩增的模板。

(1) 采外周血 0.2 mL 于含有 EDTA 抗凝剂的 1.5 mL 的微量离心管中。

(2) 加 1 mL RBC 裂解缓冲液于样品中,轻轻混匀。

(3) 离心 4 000 r/min,3 min,弃上清。微量离心管底部可见白细胞层。

(4) 重复(2)和(3)三次,最后一次用卫生纸吸干管壁的液体,注意别碰上白细胞层。

(5) 加 100 μL WBC 裂解缓冲液于白细胞层,混匀,裂解 WBC。

(6) 将微量离心管放于 60℃水中水浴 30 min。

(7) 再将微量离心管放入沸水中煮 3~5 min,以便灭活蛋白酶 K。

(8) 以 1 000 r/min 离心 2 min,取上清中即含有 DNA,用做 PCR 扩增的模板。

2. PCR 扩增 HLA－B27 基因:应用 HLA－B27 基因的序列特异性引物(SSP)与样品中 HLA－B27 基因互补结合,经 PCR 扩增 HLA－B27 基因。

(1) 吸取 2 μL DNA(约 60 ng)模板于含有 PCR 混合液的 PCR 小管中,混匀。注意,不要将 DNA 模板加入矿物油层。

(2)PCR 循环

预变性	94℃	2 min	
变性	94℃	45 s	×10 个循环
退火	65℃	75 s	
变性	94℃	45 s	
退火	61℃	1 min	×20 个循环
延伸	72℃	45 s	

3. 琼脂糖凝胶电泳检测 *HLA-B27* DNA 片段：将 PCR 产物进行琼脂糖凝胶电泳，如果凝胶中有条带，提示样品为 *HLA-B27*(+)；如果凝胶中无条带，提示样品为 *HLA-B27*(-)。

(1)吸取 20 μL PCR 产物于凝胶的点样孔中。

(2)用 160 V 的电压电泳 20 min。

(3)在紫外灯下观察结果并拍照。

【结果】

图 9-5 显示：

如果凝胶中有 PCR 产物，提示样品为 *HLA-B27*(+)。

如果凝胶中无 PCR 产物，提示样品为 *HLA-B27*(-)。

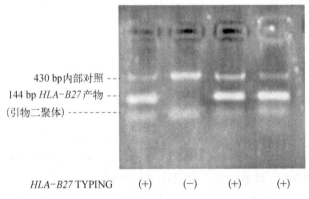

430 bp内部对照 --
144 bp *HLA-B27* 产物 --
(引物二聚体) ---------

HLA-B27 TYPING　　(+)　　(-)　　(+)　　(+)

图 9-5 *HLA-B27*(+)样品中 *HLA-B27* 特异性条带

【注意事项】

1. 由于 PCR-SSP 技术对污染的 DNA 较为敏感，加样时应防止污染。

2. 凝胶电泳时使用的 DNA 染料(溴化乙锭)是致突变剂，操作时应戴手套，废液或废物应妥善处理。

【思考题】

试述 SSP-PCR 技术检测 *HLA-B27* 基因的原理。

(尹丙姣　吴雄文)

Exp. 9   HLA Typing for *B27* with PCR – SSP

【Principle】

The genes encoding for *HLA* are the most polymorphic in human genome, i. e. many alleles at each locus in a random population. Each allele has its own unique DNA sequences, which is the molecular basis for HLA DNA typing.

HLA allele sequence specific primers (SSP) are designed to bind to the corresponding HLA allele sequences complimentarily. The specific complementary binding of a pair of given primers to the sample DNA will result in the amplification of the DNA fragment by PCR. The presence of the PCR product indicates the sample DNA bearing the corresponding *HLA* allele and the primer is designed to bind to. The following figures are the flow chart of *HLA* – *B27* typing by PCR – SSP(Fig.9 – 1 – Fig.9 – 4).

whole blood sample
↓
RBC lysis, harvest nucleated cells
↓
digestion with proteinase K, DNA is released from nuclei
↓
DNA is resolved in aqueous phase, and used as PCR template
↓
PCR amplification with *HLA* – *B27* sequence specific primer (SSP)
↓
agarose gel electrophoresis check for PCR product
↓
if PCR product is present, the sample is typed as *HLA* – *B27* (+)
if PCR product is absent, the sample is typed as *HLA* – *B27* (–)

Fig.9 – 1   Flow chart of *HLA* – *B27* typing by PCR – SSP

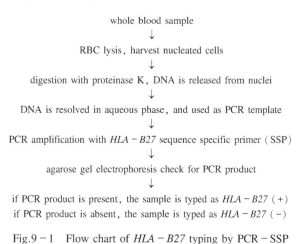

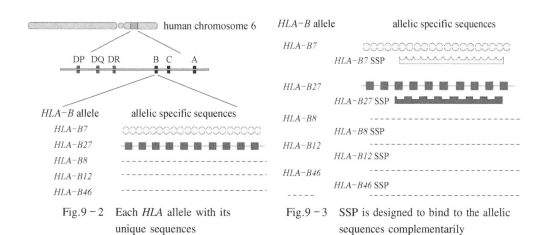

Fig.9 – 2   Each *HLA* allele with its unique sequences

Fig.9 – 3   SSP is designed to bind to the allelic sequences complementarily

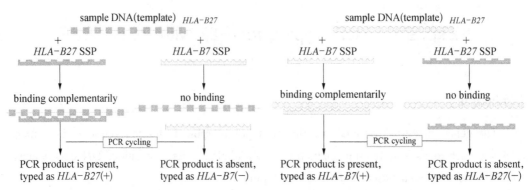

Fig.9 - 4　Sequence-specific primer is used to type *HLA* allele with PCR

【Application】

1. Tissue typing for allogeneic transplantation.

2. Study for HLA related diseases.

3. Forensic medicine, anthropology.

【Materials】

1. Blood sample, 0. 2 mL EDTA whole blood in 1. 5 mL microcentrifuge tube, with known *HLA - B27* type

2. RBC lysis buffer

3. WBC lysis buffer

4. PCR mixture

5. Loading buffer(cresol red,final concentration 0. 001%, *m/V*)

6. Centrifuge tube, pipette, centrifuge, PCR machine, etc.

【Procedures】

1. The DNA samples as the template for PCR reaction is extracted from WBC:

(1) Collect 0. 2 mL peripheral blood in a 1. 5 mL microcentrifuge tube with anti-agglutination with EDTA.

(2) Add 1 mL RBC-lysis buffer to the samples, and mix gently.

(3) Spin down the tube with 4,000 r/min, 3 min. Discard the supernatant, WBC layer can be seen at the bottom of the tube.

(4) Repeat step (2) and (3) for 3 times. Using tissue (or a cotton stick) to dry the liquid drops on the wall of the tube. Be careful not to touch the WBC layer.

(5) Add 100 μL WBC lysis buffer to the tube containing WBC layer. Mix well to disperse the WBC.

(6) Incubate the tube at 60℃ water bath for 30 min.

(7) Put the tube into the boiling water bath for 3 − 5 min, to inactivate the proteinase K.

(8) Centrifuge the tube with 1,000 r/min for 2 min, the supernatant is the DNA-containing solution, which is used for the PCR template.

2. PCR amplification for *HLA* − *B27*: *HLA* − *B27* allele sequence specific primers (SSP) is used to amplify a fragment of *HLA* −*B27* allele by PCR reaction. This *HLA* − *B27* SSP is able to bind the *HLA* − *B27* allele sequences complimentarily. Amplify the corresponding fragment during PCR cycling.

(1) Pipet 2 μL DNA (about 60 ng) template and transfer it into a tube containing PCR mixture.

Caution: do not add the DNA template into the mineral oil layer.

(2) PCR cycling

Pre-denature	94℃	2 min	
Denature	94℃	45 s	×10 cycles
Anneal	65℃	75 s	
Denature	94℃	45 s	
Anneal	61℃	1 min	×20 cycles
Extension	72℃	45 s	

3. Agarose gel electrophoresis for check *HLA* − *B27* fragment: PCR product is checked with agarose gel electrophoresis. In this experiment, if the PCR product is present, the sample is typed as *HLA* − *B27*(+); if the PCR product is absent, the sample is typed as *HLA* − *B27*(−).

(1) Suck 20 μL PCR product (the orange part in the tube), and load into a well of agarose gel.

(2) Run the gel for 20 min, set V = 160 V.

(3) Check the gel under UV light. Take photos if necessary.

【Results】

Results shown in Fig.9 − 5:

If PCR product is present, the sample is typed as *HLA* − *B27* (+)

If PCR product is absent, the sample is typed as *HLA* − *B27* (−)

【Precautions】

1. Due to the high sensitivity of the PCR − SSP technique, please take care to avoid the cross-pollution when the DNA template is sucked and transferred into a tube containing PCR mixture.

2. The dye for DNA staining (ethidium bromide) is a kind of carcinogen. Please be careful to dispose it properly, and avoid its pollution.

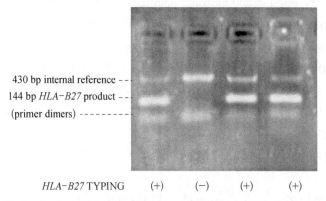

430 bp internal reference - -
144 bp *HLA-B27* product - -
(primer dimers) - - - - - - - -

HLA-B27 TYPING   (+)   (−)   (+)   (+)

Fig.9 − 5   Specific bands can be seen with *HLA − B27*(+) samples

【Question】

Please explain the principle of the *HLA* typing for *B27* with PCR − SSP.

(Yin Bingjiao   Wu Xiongwen)

第二篇
Chapter Two

免疫细胞分离
Isolation of Immune Cells

2.1

免疫细胞的分离和纯化
Separation and Purification of Immune Cells

实验十　外周血单个核细胞分离

【原理】

人外周血单个核细胞分离的常用方法之一是葡聚糖—泛影葡胺密度梯度离心法（ficoll-hypaque density gradient centrifugation）。在试管中,将血液重叠于淋巴细胞分层液（密度1.077 g/L）之上离心时,由于粒细胞（1.090 g/L）、红细胞（1.092 g/L）、淋巴细胞（1.070 g/L）的密度不同而相互分开。从顶部到底部可分为四层:血浆、单核细胞、淋巴细胞、粒白细胞及红细胞（图10-1）。

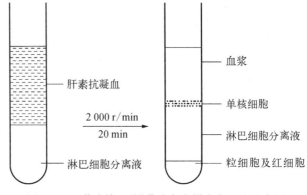

图10-1　葡聚糖-泛影葡胺密度梯度离心法示意图

【应用】

分离外周血单个核细胞,体外检测该细胞的数量和功能。

【材料】

1. 肝素溶液:500 U/mL
2. 淋巴细胞分离液:密度（1.077±0.001）g/L
3. Hank's 平衡盐溶液（HBSS:pH 7.2~7.4）
4. 0.5%台盼蓝染液
5. 注射器、离心管、试管、吸管、离心机、显微镜等

【方法】

1. 采集静脉血2 mL 注入盛有0.1 mL 肝素的试管中,混匀。
2. 加入2 mL 的 HBSS 稀释血液。
3. 取淋巴细胞分离液2 mL 加入离心管中,再将稀释血液小心地加在淋巴细胞分离液上,注意保持两界面清晰。
4. 室温下,2 000 r/min 离心20 min。
5. 用毛细吸管轻轻吸出单个核细胞层,加入含有5 mL HBSS 的试管中,混匀。
6. 1 500 r/min 离心10 min。弃上清后,再洗一次。
7. 弃上清,用 HBSS 将细胞悬液恢复至1 mL。计数细胞,将细胞悬液调至实验所需浓度。
8. 取0.1 mL 细胞悬液加0.5%台盼蓝1 滴,混匀。5~10 min 后,制压滴片。高倍镜

下计数活细胞数(未染色)和死细胞数(染成蓝色)。

【结果】

回收的细胞中单个核细胞应占 90% 以上,细胞存活率应大于 95%。

【注意事项】

1. 抽血后在 4 h 内使用。
2. 全过程在室温下进行。
3. 加血于分离液上一定要轻缓,避免破坏界面。
4. 若收集的单个核细胞用于淋巴细胞转化试验,则用 1 mL 含 5% 胎牛血清的 RPMI - 1640 保存细胞;若用于第二天的试验,则用 2 mL 含 5% 胎牛血清的 RPMI - 1640 保存细胞。

【思考题】

为什么使用葡聚糖—泛影葡胺分离液能将单个核细胞从全血中分离出来?

(刘　春　李　群)

Exp. 10 Separation of Mononuclear Cells from Whole Peripheral Blood

【Principle】

Ficoll-hypaque density gradient centrifugation is commonly used for separation of mononuclear cells from peripheral blood. In a test tube, whole peripheral blood is gently overlaid onto a lymphocyte separation medium (LSM) (with a specific gravity of 1.077) (e.g. ficoll-hypaque). Following centrifugation, lymphocytes (1.070 g/L) are separated from granulocytes (1.090 g/L) and erythrocytes (1.092 g/L) according to its specific gravity. Four distinct layers are formed from top to bottom: plasma, mononuclear cells, LSM, granulocytes and erythrocytes (Fig.10 - 1).

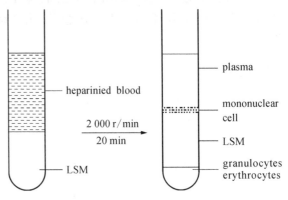

Fig.10 - 1 Ficoll-hypaque centrifugation

【Application】

Separation of PBMCs supplies a major source of lymphocytes for detecting the number and function of lymphocyte *in vitro*.

【Materials】

1. Heparin solution: 500 U/mL
2. LSM: specific gravity (1.077±0.001) g/L
3. Hank's balanced salt solution (HBSS: pH7.2 - 7.4)
4. 0.5% trypan blue solution
5. Syringes, centrifuge tube, pipette, centrifuge, microscope, etc.

【Procedures】

1. Draw 2 mL of human venous blood and mix it with 0.1 mL heparin in a test tube.
2. Dilute whole blood with an equal volume of HBSS.
3. Pipette 2 mL LSM into a centrifuge tube. Carefully overlay the LSM with diluted blood sample by slowly adding blood down the side of the tube. The surface of the LSM must not be disturbed.

4. Centrifuge at 2,000 r/min for 20 min at room temperature.

5. Use a pipette, discard the plasma layer and harvest the mononuclear band from tube at the interface between the plasma and LSM gradient. Transfer to a test tube containing 5 mL HBSS. Mix well.

6. Centrifuge at 1,500 r/min for 10 min. Discard supernatant and repeat step.

7. Resuspend the cell button in 1 mL HBSS. Perform cell count and adjust cell suspension to desired cell concentration.

8. Add a drop of 0.5% trypan blue to the tube containing 0.1 mL of cell suspension. Mix well. After 5 – 10 min, add a drop of the mixture to the slide and put a cover glass. Count the viable (unstained) and dead cells (stained) under the microscope.

【Results】

Over 90% of cells obtained by this means are mononuclear cells. The viability of cells is over 95%.

【Precautions】

1. Blood must be used after 4 h of collection.

2. All processes are made at room temperature.

3. Gently and slowly overlay the LSM with the blood sample. Avoid destroy the surfaces.

4. If the cells are used for lymphocyte transformation assays, resuspend in 1 mL RPMI – 1640 with 5% fetal calf serum. If the cells are to be held overnight for testing the following day, add 2 mL RPMI – 1640 with 5% fetal calf serum and store them at room temperature.

【Question】

Why can Ficoll-Hypaque medium separate mononuclear cells from whole peripheral blood?

(Liu Chun   Li Qun)

实验十一　　小鼠骨髓来源巨噬细胞制备

【原理】

骨髓来源的巨噬细胞(BMDM)是原代巨噬细胞,是骨髓细胞在生长因子存在下体外培养而来的。巨噬细胞集落刺激因子(M－CSF)是谱系特异性生长因子,能促进髓样祖细胞增殖和分化成巨噬细胞/单核细胞谱系的细胞。一旦分化,贴壁的巨噬细胞与悬浮生长的其他细胞分离。BMDM适用于多种类型的实验操作,包括形态学、基因表达和生理学研究。例如,巨噬细胞具有摄取微生物的独特能力。

【应用】

培养原代巨噬细胞,并用于巨噬细胞功能分析,如吞噬功能检测、巨噬细胞极化分析等。

【材料】

1. 小鼠(6~8周龄)
2. RPMI－1640培养液
3. DMEM培养液(包含10%胎牛血清)
4. M－CSF
5. LPS(脂多糖)
6. 细胞因子(鼠源性):IFN－γ、IL-4、IL－13
7. 红细胞裂解液 AKT(NH$_4$Cl 150 mmol/L, KHCO$_3$ 10 mmol/L, Na$_2$EDTA 0.1 mmol/L)
8. 200目的无菌钢丝网、吸管、剪刀、镊子、注射器、离心机,75%乙醇,细胞刮

【方法】

1. 颈椎脱臼处死小鼠。处死小鼠后,用剪刀除去腿骨上面的肌肉组织,然后剪断骨头两端的肌腱使其游离。无菌条件下取股骨、胫骨。用75%乙醇消毒骨头,并用RPMI－1640培养液冲洗(图11－1)。

2. 剪开股骨或胫骨两端,用注射器吸取RPMI－1640培养基冲洗出骨髓腔中的骨髓细胞,4℃离心5 min,1 600 r/min。弃上清,用AKT去除红细胞,用预冷的RPMI－1640培养基洗两遍,4℃离心5 min,1 600 r/min。最后用细胞计数板计数,用DMEM培养基将细胞浓度调整为2×10^{6}个/mL。

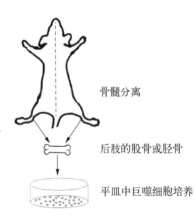

骨髓分离

后肢的股骨或胫骨

平皿中巨噬细胞培养

图11－1　小鼠骨髓来源巨噬细胞分离流程图

3. 按照所需铺板,如只需六孔板中的 3 个孔,则取 $6×10^6$ 个细胞重悬到终体积为 6 mL 的 DMEM 培养基(即每孔 2 mL),再加入 20 ng/mL 的 M-CSF。

4. 3 天后,可见大量巨噬细胞贴壁。吸取上清悬浮细胞,在每个孔中直接加入预热的 DMEM 培养基和 30~50 ng/mL M-CSF。

5. 37℃孵育 3 天,获得的巨噬细胞为 M0,弃掉培养上清,每孔加入 DMEM 培养基,用细胞刮轻轻刮取细胞,计数。计数后的巨噬细胞如果重新铺板,需要贴壁 2 h,相关刺激应在贴壁之后再进行。

6. 如需诱导成 M1 或 M2,可弃掉上清,加入 100 ng/mL LPS 和 20 ng/mL IFN-γ 诱导 2 天后,即为 M1;或加入 20 ng/mL IL-4 和 20 ng/mL IL-13 诱导 2 天后,即为 M2。

【结果】

贴壁的巨噬细胞应占 50% 以上。

【注意事项】

1. 整个过程保持无菌操作。
2. 巨噬细胞贴壁牢固,细胞刮使用要轻柔。

【思考题】

如果分离的巨噬细胞比例偏低,请分析可能的影响因素。

（周媛媛　章晓联）

Exp. 11　Preparation of Mouse Bone Marrow-Derived Macrophages

【Principle】

Bone marrow-derived macrophages (BMDM) are primary macrophage cells, derived from bone marrow cells *in vitro* in the presence of growth factors. Macrophage colony-stimulating factor (M－CSF) is a lineage-specific growth factor that is responsible for the proliferation and differentiation of committed myeloid progenitors into cells of the macrophage/monocyte lineage. Once differentiated, the adherent macrophages can be separated from other cells grown in suspension. And BMDMs are used for various types of experimental manipulations, including morphological, gene expression, and physiological studies. For example, macrophages have the unique ability to ingest microbes.

【Application】

To culture primary macrophage and analyze the functions of macrophages, such as to determine the phagocytosis function or polarization of macrophages.

【Materials】

1. Mice (6－8 weeks old)
2. RPMI－1640 medium
3. DMEM medium (containing 10% fetal bovine serum, streptomycin, penicillin)
4. M－CSF
5. Lipopolysaccharides (LPS)
6. Cytokines (murine): IFN－γ, IL-4, IL－13
7. AKT (NH$_4$Cl 150 mmol/L, KHCO$_3$ 10 mmol/L, Na$_2$EDTA 0.1 mmol/L)
8. Sterilized stainless steel screen (200 mesh), pipettes, scissors, forceps, centrifuge, syringe, 75% alcohol, cell scraper

【Procedures】

1. Sacrifice mouse by cervical dislocation. After sacrificing mouse cut the skin, use scissors to remove all muscle tissues from the bones of legs. Cut the tendon of bones at both ends to release them. The femur and tibia are taken under aseptic conditions. Sterilize the bones with 75% ethanol, wash the bones with RPMI－1640 medium (Fig.11－1).

2. Cut off both ends of the bones, flush the bone marrow-derived cells in the bones with RPMI－1640 medium by syringe. Centrifuge at 1,600 r/min at 4℃ for 5 min. Discard the

supernatant, remove red blood cells with AKT, take pre-cooled RPMI－1640 medium and wash it 2 times. Centrifuge at 1,600 r/min for 5 min at 4℃. Finally, count the bone marrow-derived cells using a hemacytometer. Adjust the concentration to 2×10^6 cells/mL in DMEM medium.

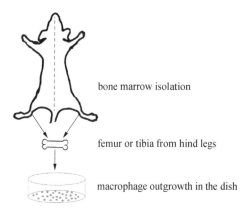

bone marrow isolation

femur or tibia from hind legs

macrophage outgrowth in the dish

Fig.11－1   Schematic diagram of isolation of bone marrow-derived macrophages

3. Plate the cells. If only 3 wells of six-wells plates are needed, take 6×10^6 cells. Resuspend to a final volume of 6 mL DMEM medium (2 mL per well, 2×10^6 cells/well) and add 20 ng/mL M－CSF.

4. After 3 days, a large number of macrophages can adhere to the wall of well plates. Aspirate the supernatant, then add the pre-warmed DMEM medium and 30－50 ng/mL M－CSF to each well.

5. After incubate at 37℃ for 3 days, the obtained macrophages are M0. Discard the culture supernatant, add DMEM medium to each well, and scrape the cells gently with a cell scraper, then count cells. If the counted macrophages are re-plated, it takes 2 hours to adhere, and the relevant stimulation should be done after it.

6. If the macrophages are needed to be induced into M1 or M2. Add 100 ng/ml LPS and 20 ng/ml IFN－γ and incubate cells for two days. Macrophages can be induced as M1; or add 20 ng/ml IL-4 and 20 ng/ml IL－13 and incubate cells for two days, they can be induced as M2.

【Results】

Adherent macrophages should be over 50%.

【Precautions】

1. Keep sterility throughout the entire procedure.

2. Since macrophages adhere firmly to the well, we should use cell scrapers carefully and gently.

【Question】

If the ratio of macrophages isolated is low, please analyze the possible reasons?

(Zhou Yuanyuan   Zhang Xiaolian)

实验十二　　小鼠腹腔巨噬细胞的分离

【原理】

腹腔巨噬细胞来源于造血干细胞(骨髓干细胞)。在骨髓中,造血干细胞经前单核细胞分化为单核细胞,之后进入血液,随着血流到达腹腔成为巨噬细胞。巨噬细胞作为免疫系统中重要的免疫细胞之一,在免疫应答中发挥重要作用。腹腔巨噬细胞具有吞噬作用、杀伤肿瘤作用、特异性免疫中的抗原提呈作用,以及激活和调节免疫应答等各种功能。

直接收集小鼠的腹腔巨噬细胞获得的数量较少,因此可以先于小鼠腹腔中注射刺激剂(4%巯基乙酸肉汤),诱导巨噬细胞渗出,然后收集腹腔渗出液中的巨噬细胞。

【应用】

获取小鼠腹腔巨噬细胞,用于巨噬细胞的吞噬功能检测等功能研究。

【材料】

1. 小鼠(约6周龄)
2. 4%巯基乙酸肉汤
3. RPMI－1640培养液
4. DMEM培养基
5. PBS－H(含10 U/mL肝素和10%小牛血清的PBS)
6. 0.4%台盼蓝染色液、吸管、剪刀、镊子、离心机、注射器、75%乙醇

【方法】

1. 剃去小鼠腹部的毛并用75%乙醇消毒。腹腔注射5 mL的4%(m/V)巯基乙酸肉汤。3~4天后收集腹腔细胞。如要收集腹腔静置巨噬细胞,不注射刺激物,直接从第2步开始(图12－1)。

2. 消毒腹部,沿腹中线注入2 mL预冷的无菌PBS－H。轻轻按摩腹部1 min。

3. 以下均无菌操作。剪开腹壁,用镊子夹起皮肤,用吸管吸出渗出液,再用同样容量的预冷PBS－H冲洗

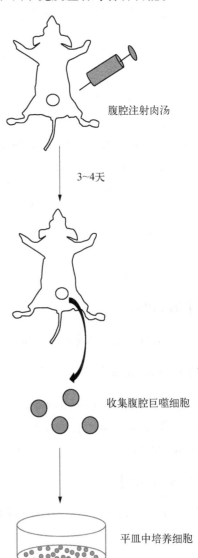

腹腔注射肉汤

3~4天

收集腹腔巨噬细胞

平皿中培养细胞

图12－1　分离腹腔巨噬细胞流程示意图

腹腔 2~3 次。合并渗出液于离心管中,4℃离心10 min。弃上清液。

4. 用预冷的 RPMI－1640 培养液洗涤细胞 3 次,每次 4℃、1 600 r/min 离心 10 min。弃上清液。用预冷的 RPMI－1640 培养液悬浮细胞。

5. 将分离的细胞按照 $2 \times 10^5 \sim 4 \times 10^5$ 个/mL 接种于培养皿中,在 5% CO_2 培养箱中 37℃孵育 24 h。

6. 轻轻晃动培养皿,弃细胞上清,用预冷的 PBS 洗一次。用细胞刮刮下细胞,轻轻吹打使细胞分散均匀。

7. 用预冷的 PBS－H 洗涤收集的细胞 3 次,每次 4℃、1 600 r/min 离心 10 min。

8. 重新加入 RPMI－1640 培养液重悬细胞,配成所需浓度的巨噬细胞悬液。台盼蓝染色计数细胞存活率。

【结果】

使用细胞计数板计数,并分析分离的腹腔巨噬细胞活性。

【注意事项】

1. 整个操作过程注意保持无菌。
2. 破碎红细胞过程要轻柔。
3. 巨噬细胞贴壁牢固,使用细胞刮子要小心,不要导致过多细胞碎片。
4. 检测细胞存活率的步骤不能省略,活细胞数过低会影响实验的正常进行。

【思考题】

如果分离的细胞中巨噬细胞比例偏低,请分析可能的影响因素。

(姚琪利　谢　焱　章晓联)

Exp. 12   Isolation of Mouse Peritoneal Macrophages

【Principle】

Peritoneal macrophages are derived from hematopoietic stem cells (bone marrow stem cells). In the bone marrow, hematopoietic stem cells differentiate into pre-monocytes, then into mononuclear cells before entering the bloodstream. When reaching the peritoneal cavity with the blood flow, mononuclear cells further differentiate into macrophages. Macrophages, as one of the important immune cells in the immune system, play important roles in immune responses. Peritoneal macrophages possess multiple functions such as phagocytosis, anti-tumor effect, antigen presentation in adaptive immunity, and activation / regulation of immune responses.

The amount of peritoneal macrophages obtained through direct harvesting from mouse peritoneal cavity is limited. Thus, thioglycollate elicitation (injection of 4% brewer thioglycollate medium into the peritoneal cavity) is usually applied to induce exudation of macrophages, and increase the amount of macrophages from peritoneal exudate.

【Application】

Harvest mouse peritoneal macrophages for further study, including evaluation of the phagocytic function of macrophages.

【Materials】

1. Mice (about 6 weeks old)
2. 4% brewer thioglycollate medium
3. RPMI − 1640 medium
4. DMEM medium
5. PBS − H (phosphate buffered saline containing 10 U/mL heparin and 10% calf serum)
6. 0.4% trypan blue staining solution, pipettes, scissors, forceps, centrifuge, syringe, 75% alcohol

【Procedures】

1. The mouse abdomen was shaved and disinfect with 75% alcohol. Inject 5 mL of 4% (m/V) brewer thioglycollate medium into the peritoneal cavity of each mouse and harvest peritoneal macrophages 3 − 4 days later. If you want to collect unstimulated peritoneal macrophages, skip this step and start directly from Step 2 (Fig.12 − 1).

2. Disinfect the abdomen with 75% alcohol. Inject 2 mL pre-cooled sterile PBS − H

along the midline of the abdomen. Gently massage the abdomen for 1 min.

3. Strict aseptic techniques should be used for the following steps. Make an incision in the skin of the peritoneum while holding up the skin with a pair of forceps. Use a pipette to collect the exudate from the cavity. Rinse the abdominal cavity 2 − 3 times with the same volume of pre-cooled PBS − H. Combine the exudate in a single centrifuge tube. Centrifuge at 1 600 r/min, 4℃ for 10 min. Discard the supernatant.

4. Wash the cells three times with pre-cooled RPMI − 1640 medium by centrifugation at 1 600 r/min, 4℃ for 10 min. Discard the supernatant. Resuspend the cells in pre-cooled RPMI − 1640 medium.

5. Seed the isolated cells into a Petri dish to $(2-4) \times 10^5$ cells/mL and incubate for 24 h at 37℃ in a 5% CO_2 incubator.

6. Gently rock the dish. Discard the cell supernatant, and wash once with pre-cooled PBS. Scrape the cells with cells scraper, and spread the cells evenly through gentle blowing.

7. Wash the collected cells 3 times with pre-cooled PBS − H by centrifugation at 1 600 r/min, 4℃ for 10 min.

8. Re-suspend the cells in RPMI − 1640 medium. Adjust cell suspension to desired concentration. Assess cell viability by trypan blue staining.

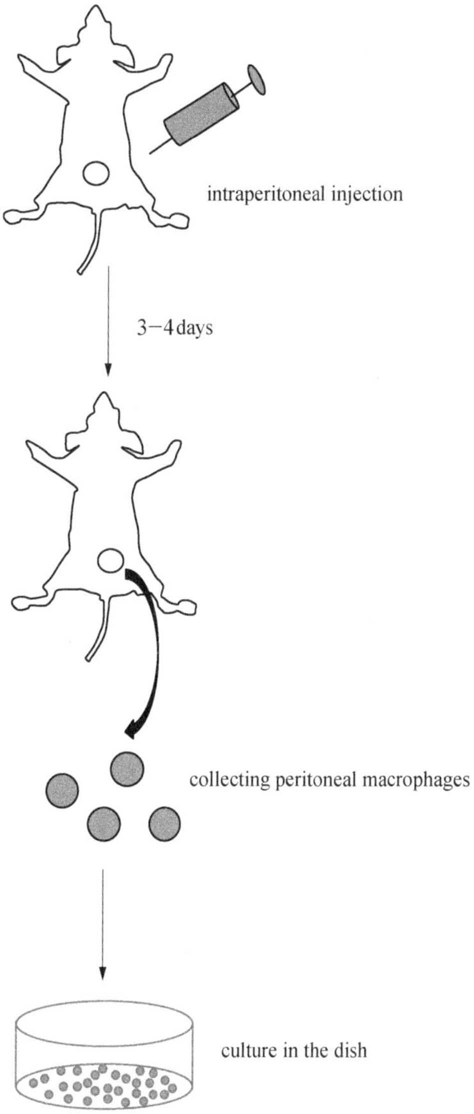

intraperitoneal injection

3−4 days

collecting peritoneal macrophages

culture in the dish

Fig.12 − 1　Schematic diagram of isolation of peritoneal macrophages

【Results】

The viable cells are counted using a cell counting plate, and the isolated peritoneal macrophages are subjected to cell activity analysis.

【Precautions】

1. Strict aseptic techniques should be used throughout the entire procedure.
2. The process of disrupting red blood cells should be gentle.

3. Macrophages adhere firmly to the well. Use cell scrapers carefully, and do not cause excessive cell debris.

4. The step of assessing cell viability cannot be omitted, and scarcity of viable cells will affect the normal conduct of the experiment.

【Question】

If the percentage of macrophages in the isolated cells is low, please analyze the possible reasons.

(Yao Qili   Xie Yan   Zhang Xiaolian)

实验十三　　树突状细胞的制备

【原理】

树突状细胞(DC)是体内功能最强的专职抗原提呈细胞,可把抗原特异性地提呈给 T 淋巴细胞而产生抗原特异性免疫应答。

根据实验需要,可分别利用小鼠或人的多种标本,在体外制备 DC。本实验介绍从人外周血中制备 DC 的方法。DC 占人外周血单个核细胞总数的 0.5%～1.0%,从外周血中制备 DC,需先从外周血中分离、获得单个核细胞,然后,可用贴壁法继续获得单核细胞,经 GM-CSF 和 IL-4 两种细胞因子共同诱导,就可获得 DC。GM-CSF 可促进 DC 增殖,IL-4 则可抑制巨噬细胞增生而利于干细胞向 DC 分化。

目前尚未发现 DC 的特异性标记,国内外鉴定 DC 主要采用 CD1a 和 CD83 分子,CD1a 主要表达于人胸腺细胞、DC(包括 Langerhans 细胞),是鉴定人外周血与骨髓中 DC 的最好标记,CD83 是 DC 的成熟标记,在 DC 培养早期不表达 CD83 分子,当成熟时才表达 CD83 分子,此时 DC 激活 T 细胞功能最强。所以目前主要用 CD1a 阳性细胞的多少来反映 DC 的数量。

【应用】

研究 DC 的功能及用于过继免疫治疗。

【材料】

1. 淋巴细胞培养液
2. 500×10^6 单个核细胞
3. rhIL-3、GM-CSF 和 rhIL-4
4. 5 mmol/L EDTA 四钠盐,以 PBS 配制,除菌过滤,使用前预温到 37℃
5. 175 cm² 组织培养瓶,50 mL 锥底离心管,Sorvall RT-6000B 离心机及 H-1000 转子
6. 台盼蓝溶液、异硫氰酸荧光素 FITC-CD1a 单抗及流式细胞计数仪等

【方法】

1. 贴壁法获得单核细胞。

(1) 取 20 mL、预热至 37℃ 的淋巴细胞培养液,加入到 175 cm² 的组织培养瓶内,37℃ 孵育 30 min。

(2) 取含有 500×10^6 单个核细胞的 10 mL 淋巴细胞培养液到上述培养瓶中,同时加入 rhIL-3 至终浓度为 200 U/mL。

(3) 37℃ 孵育 3 h,每小时轻轻摇动培养瓶一次。

(4) 用吸管吸去培养液及其中未贴壁的细胞。用 20 mL、37℃ 的淋巴细胞培养液洗

贴壁细胞两次。

2. 制备 DC。

(1) 取含有 800 U/mL GM-CSF 和 1 000 U/ml rhIL-4 的 30 mL 淋巴细胞培养液到上述培养瓶内,37℃孵育,每隔 2 d,半量换液一次,补充新鲜培养液(含有 1 600 U/mL GM-CSF 和 1 000 U/mL rhIL-4,至终浓度分别为 800 U/mL 和 500 U/mL),连续 3 次。

(2) 第 7 天,移出非贴壁的细胞,置于 50 mL 的锥底离心管中,加 20 mL、5 mmol/L EDTA/PBS 到培养瓶中,37℃孵育 20 min,反复用力吹吸培养瓶内的介质,使贴壁细胞完全脱落,转移至 50 mL 锥底离心管中,与非贴壁细胞混合。

(3) 25℃以 1 500 r/min 离心 10 min,吸去上清,将沉淀重悬在适量的淋巴细胞培养液中。

【结果】

1. 细胞计数,并采用台盼蓝法分析细胞活性。
2. 用流式细胞仪检测细胞表面的 CD1a 分子,确定获得的 DC 的纯度。

【注意事项】

通过用含有血清的培养液和 IL-3 对培养瓶进行预处理,可提高单核细胞的产量,需注意的是 IL-3 对非贴壁的淋巴细胞会有一定影响;也可通过免疫磁珠技术等方法获得不含淋巴细胞的外周血细胞。

【思考题】

请说出一种用 DC 进行过继免疫治疗的方法、原理及临床意义。

(何金生)

Exp. 13 Generation Isolation of Dendritic Cells

【Principle】

Dendritic cells (DC) are the most potent antigen presenting cell (APC) known, which have numerous specialized features that make them extremely efficient at capturing and presenting antigen, activating T cells and mediating immune response.

DCs can be generated and isolated, *in vitro*, from many different samples of human beings or mice in different experiments. Generation and isolation of DCs from the human peripheral blood is one of many methods. DCs only constitute 0.5%−1.0% of the peripheral blood mononuclear cells. To generate this cell population, the first step is to isolate monocytes from the peripheral blood by exploiting the adherence property of monocytes.

DCs can be generated from the monocyte population by differentiation in the presence of rhIL-4 and Granulocyte/Macrophage Colony Stimulating Factor (GM-CSF). The rhIL-4 is used to suppress macrophages overgrowth. The addition of GM-CSF promotes DC proliferation.

Many surface markers are not rigorously DC-specific, but they are still useful in identifying DCs. These include CD83 and CD1a molecules. CD1a molecules present on cortical thymocytes, DCs and a subset of B-cells. DCs can be distinguished from monocytes/macrophages by the presence of cell-surface CD1a molecules. The CD83 molecular is a marker for the mature DCs, which present the most powerful function to activate T cells. Therefore, the number of DCs are related with the more or less of CD1a positive cell.

【Application】

DCs can be used as the research tool of functional study and adoptive immune therapy.

【Materials】

1. Lymphocyte culture medium (LCM)

2. 500×10^6 PBMC population

3. Recombinant human interleukin 3 (rhIL-3), interleukin 4 (rhIL-4), and GM-CSF

4. 5 mmol/L tetrasodium EDTA in PBS, filter-sterilized using 0.22 μm filter, prewarmed to 37℃

5. 175 cm² tissue culture flasks, 50 mL conical centrifuge tubes, Sorvall RT-6000B centrifuge with H-1000 rotor (or equivalent)

6. Trypan blue, FITC-CD1a mAb and flow cytometry, etc.

【Procedures】

1. Allow monocyte population to attach to plastic dish

(1) Add 20 mL of 37℃ LCM to 175 cm² tissue culture flasks. Incubate LCM for 30 min.

(2) Add 500×10^6 PBMC in 10 mL LCM to each flask plus rhIL-3 to a final concentration of 200 U/mL.

(3) Incubate for 3 h, gently rock flasks every hour.

(4) Remove nonadherent cells by aspirating the medium. Wash flasks twice, each time with 20 mL LCM with 37℃.

2. Isolate DC

(1) Add 30 mL LCM. GM-CSF and rhIL-4 are added at final concentrations of 800 and 1,000 U/mL, respectively. Cultures are fed every other day (days 2, 4, and 6) by removing 15 mL of the medium and adding back 15 mL fresh medium with cytokines (1,600 U/mL GM-CSF and 1,000 U/mL rhIL-4, resulting in final concentrations of 800 and 500 U/mL, respectively).

(2) On day 7, remove nonadherent cells and place them in 50 mL centrifuge tubes, then add 20 mL of 5 mmol/L EDTA/PBS to each flask and incubate for 20 min to release adherent cells. Vigorously pipet medium up and down to detach adherent cells, then combine with nonadherent cells in 50 mL centrifuge tubes.

(3) Centrifuge at 1,500 r/min (in Sorvall H - 1,000 rotor) at 25℃ for 10 min. Aspirate supernatant and resuspend cell pellet in LCM.

【Results】

1. Count cells and determine number of viable cells by trypan blue exclusion.

2. Test CD1a on the cell surface by flow cytometry and determine purity of the DC populations.

【Precautions】

Isolation of monocytes by adherence is significantly enhanced by precoating the tissue culture flasks with serum-containing medium and IL-3 during the adhesion incubation. However, the presence of IL-3 may influence the nonadherent lymphocytes. Additionally, the lymphocyte-depleted PBMC also can be made by means of immunomagnetic technique, etc.

【Question】

Please describe the method, principle and clinical significance of DC adoptive immune therapy.

(He Jinsheng)

实验十四　自然杀伤细胞分离

【原理】

自然杀伤(NK)细胞有重要的抗感染和抗肿瘤作用。NK细胞占人外周血淋巴细胞总数的10%~15%,占小鼠脾淋巴细胞的2.5%。分离人外周血中的NK细胞和小鼠脾脏中的NK细胞常分为两步:第一步,利用密度梯度离心法获得主要成分为淋巴细胞和单核细胞的外周血单个核细胞(PBMC)。原理:利用密度为(1.077±0.001) g/L 的 Ficoll-Hypaque 溶液作密度梯度离心时,红细胞、粒细胞密度较大(1.092 g/L 左右),离心后沉于管底;人 PBMC 密度(1.075 g/L 左右)接近 Ficoll 液,离心后位于 Ficoll 液界面(图14-1A)。第二步,利用磁珠分选试剂盒分选出 PBMC 中的 NK 细胞。原理:PBMC 中非 NK细胞(如 T 细胞、B 细胞)与生物素标记的"鸡尾酒"抗体及 NK 细胞磁珠孵育后被磁分离去除,从而获得高纯度 NK 细胞(图14-1B)。分离小鼠脾脏中的 NK 细胞,可将分散后的脾细胞直接进行磁珠分选(图14-1B)。

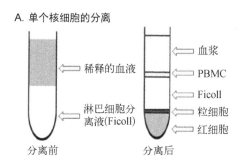

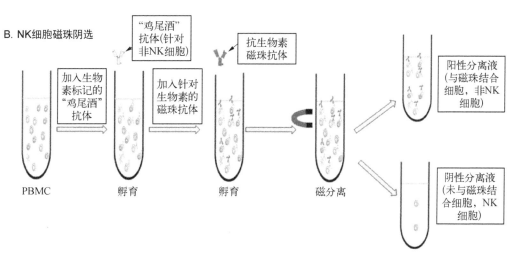

图 14-1　NK 细胞的分离

【应用】

分离人外周血 NK 细胞或小鼠脾脏 NK 细胞。

【材料】

1. 分离人外周血 NK 细胞:

(1) 健康人外周血 2 mL

(2) EDTA 抗凝管

(3) Ficoll-Hypaque 分离液

(4) RPMI－1640 完全培养基(含 10%小牛血清)

(5) 磷酸盐缓冲液(PBS)

(6) NK 细胞磁珠分选试剂盒

(7) 磁珠缓冲液(磁珠分选用)

(8) 合适的磁珠分选器和磁柱

(9) 人 NK 细胞相关流式抗体:FITC 抗人 CD3、APC 抗人 CD56

(10) 离心管、计数板、微量加样器

(11) 超净工作台、CO_2 孵箱

(12) 离心机、显微镜、流式细胞仪

2. 分离小鼠脾脏 NK 细胞:

(1) 6~8 周龄,雌性 C57BL/6 小鼠

(2) 红细胞裂解液

(3) 40 μm 尼龙滤网

(4) RPMI－1640 完全培养基(含 10%小牛血清)

(5) PBS

(6) 小鼠 NK 细胞磁珠分选试剂盒

(7) 磁珠缓冲液(磁珠分选用)

(8) 合适的磁珠分选器和磁柱

(9) 小鼠 NK 细胞相关流式抗体:FITC 抗鼠 CD3、APC 抗鼠 NK1. 1

(10) 离心管、计数板、微量加样器

(11) 超净工作台;CO_2 孵箱

(12) 离心机、流式细胞仪、显微镜

【方法】

分离人外周血 NK 细胞

1. PBMC 的分离:

(1) 静脉取血 2 mL 于 EDTA 抗凝管中。

(2) 加入 2 mL PBS 到 15 mL 离心管中,与血液充分混匀。

(3) 取一支新的 15 mL 离心管,加入 4 mL Ficoll 液。

（4）缓慢地加入稀释后的血液,加入过程中确保两种液体分层清晰。

（5）室温下 2 000 r/min 离心 30 min,升速 4,降速 2。

（6）离心后,管内分为多层。Ficoll 液上界面处为富含 PBMC 的白色云雾状狭窄带（图 14-1A）。

（7）将毛细吸管轻轻插到白色云雾层,吸出该层细胞,置入另一支无菌 15 mL 离心管中,加入 PBS 室温洗涤细胞 2~3 次,每次以 1 500 r/min 离心 5 min。

（8）离心完成后,加入 1 mL RPMI-1640,重悬细胞并计数。

2. NK 细胞磁珠阴选:

（1）确定 PBMC 数目,加入适量磁珠缓冲液,4℃、1 500 r/min 离心 5 min。

（2）每 10^7 个细胞加入 40 μL 缓冲液重悬细胞。

（3）每 10^7 个细胞加入 10 μL NK 细胞生物素标记的"鸡尾酒"抗体,混合均匀,2~8℃孵育 5 min。

（4）每 10^7 个细胞加入 30 μL 缓冲液。

（5）每 10^7 个细胞加入 20 μL NK 细胞磁珠,混合均匀,2~8℃孵育 10 min。

（6）将 MS 柱放在合适的磁珠分选器上（磁珠标记细胞不超过 10^7 选用 MS 柱,标记细胞不超过 10^8 选用 LS 柱）。

（7）适量缓冲液洗柱 1 次（MS: 500 μL; LS: 3 mL）。

（8）细胞悬液过柱,收集流出的细胞悬液。

（9）重复（7）两次,收集流出来的组分（含未标记细胞,主要为 NK 细胞）。

（10）4℃、1 500 r/min 离心 5 min,洗涤流出的悬液两次。

（11）1 mL RPMI-1640 完全培养基重悬细胞颗粒。

（12）细胞计数,部分细胞用于流式检测 NK 细胞纯度。

分离小鼠脾脏 NK 细胞

1. 脾细胞的获得:

（1）颈椎脱臼处死小鼠,完全浸没于 75% 乙醇中 10 min。小鼠俯卧位固定于板上,剪开左侧背部皮肤,暴露脾脏。无菌取脾并放入平皿中。

（2）将脾放在 40 μm 尼龙滤网上,加入 2 mL RPMI-1640 完全培养基,用注射器柱平端将脾磨碎,收集细胞悬液于 50 mL 离心管。

（3）细胞悬液 1 500 r/min 4℃离心 5 min, 弃上清,PBS 重悬沉淀,并采用相同条件离心洗涤一次。

（4）1 mL 红细胞裂解液重悬细胞,室温裂解 2 min。

（5）加入 1 mL 完全培养基终止裂解,1 500 r/min 4℃离心 5 min 弃上清,得沉淀。

（6）PBS 洗涤两次。

（7）沉淀溶于 1 mL RPMI-1640 完全培养中,细胞计数。

2. NK 细胞磁珠阴选:

（1）确定脾细胞数目,加入适量磁珠缓冲液,4℃、1 500 r/min 离心 5 min。

（2）每 10^7 个细胞加入 40 μL 缓冲液,重悬细胞。

（3）每 10^7 个细胞加入 10 μL NK 细胞生物素标记的"鸡尾酒"抗体,混合均匀,2~

8℃孵育 5 min。

(4) 每 10^7 个细胞加入 30 μL 缓冲液。

(5) 每 10^7 个细胞加入 20 μL 抗生物素磁珠抗体,混合均匀,2~8℃孵育 10 min。

(6) 将 LS 柱放在合适的磁珠分选器上(磁珠标记细胞不超过 $1×10^7$ 选用 MS 柱,标记细胞不超过 $1×10^8$ 选用 LS 柱)。

(7) 适量缓冲液洗柱 1 次(MS：500 μL；LS：3 mL)。

(8) 细胞悬液过柱,收集流出的细胞悬液。

(9) 重复(7)两次,收集流出的组分(含未标记细胞,主要为 NK 细胞)。

(10) 4℃、1 500 r/min 离心 5 min,洗涤流出的悬液两次。

(11) 1 mL RPMI－1640 完全培养基重悬细胞。

(12) 细胞计数,部分细胞用于流式检测 NK 细胞纯度。

【结果】

本法可分离人 PBMC 中 70%左右的 NK 细胞,得到的 NK 细胞纯度在 85%以上。

本法可分离小鼠脾脏约 65% 的 NK 细胞,得到的细胞纯度在 85%以上。

【注意事项】

1. 将稀释的抗凝血加于 Ficoll 液上时,要沿管壁缓慢加入,避免血液冲散分层液的液面。

2. 吸取富含 PBMC 的白色云雾层时,动作要轻巧,避免将白色云雾层冲散。

3. 磁珠缓冲液使用前要预冷,分选过程中细胞尽量保持低温。

4. 整个操作应尽可能快的完成,时间过长易造成细胞死亡。

5. 红细胞裂解时间不宜过长,易造成细胞死亡。

6. 一个 LS 柱最多结合 $1×10^8$ 磁珠标记的细胞,当细胞数目超过 $1×10^8$,应适当增加 LS 柱数量。

【思考题】

1. 本实验利用磁珠阴选 NK 细胞,这样做的好处有哪些?

2. 你认为决定本实验成败的关键有哪些?

(高 明 郑 芳)

Exp. 14　　Isolation of Natural Killer Cells

【Principle】

Natural killer (NK) cells play critical roles in immune defense against tumor and infection. NK cells constitute about 10% ‒ 15% of total lymphocytes in human peripheral blood and 2.5% of mouse splenic lymphocytes. In this protocol, a two-step isolation method is described to isolate human peripheral blood NK cells and mouse spleen NK cells. Firstly, peripheral blood mononuclear cell (PBMC), including lymphocyte and monocyte are separated from the blood by a density gradient centrifugation method. After centrifugated with Ficoll-Hypaque separation liquid [the density is (1.077 ± 0.001) g/L], the diluted blood sample can be divided into some layers (Fig. 14 ‒ 1A). Erythrocytes and granulocytes are located at the bottom of the tube for their larger densities (around1.092 g/L). PBMC are located at the interface of Ficoll for their similar density (around 1.075 g/L). NK cells are further selected from the PBMC by using a magnetic selection kit (Fig. 14 ‒ 1B). Non-NK

A. The isolation of peripheral blood mononuclear cells

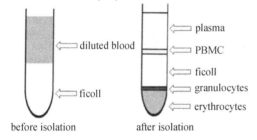

B. The negative magnetic selection of NK cells

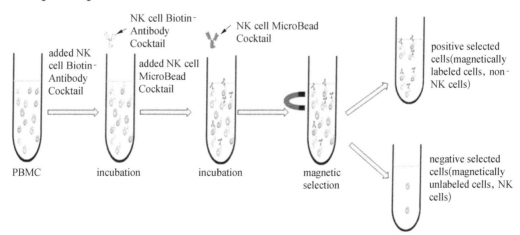

Fig. 14 ‒ 1　 Isolation of NK cells

cells, i. e. , T cells, B cells, monocytes, are magnetically labelled by using a cocktail of biotin-conjugated antibodies and the NK cell microbead cocktail. Isolation of highly pure NK cells is achieved by depletion of magnetically labeled cells. For isolation of murine natural killer cells from the spleen, the separated splenocytes are used for the negative magnetic selection of NK cells directly (Fig.14 − 1B).

【Application】

To isolate the human peripheral blood NK cells and mouse spleen NK cells.

【Materials】

1. For human peripheral blood NK cells isolation:

(1) 2 mL peripheral blood from health volunteer

(2) EDTA anti-coagulation tube

(3) Ficoll-Hypaque separation liquid

(4) Complete RPMI − 1640 culture medium (containing 10% calf serum)

(5) Phosphate buffered saline (PBS)

(6) NK Cell Isolation Kit human

(7) Bead buffer (using for magnetic selection)

(8) Suitable MACS separator and columns

(9) FITC anti-human CD3, APC anti-human CD56 (using or labeling human NK cells)

(10) Centrifugal tubes, cytometer, pipettes

(11) Super clean bench, CO_2 incubator

(12) Centrifuge, microscopes, flow cytometry

2. For mouse spleen NK cells isolation:

(1) C57/B6 mice, 6 – 8 weeks, female

(2) Red blood cell lysis buffer/ACK buffer

(3) 40 μm strainer

(4) Complete RPMI − 1640 medium (containing 10% calf serum)

(5) PBS

(6) NK Cell Isolation Kit human

(7) Bead buffer (Using for magnetic selection)

(8) Suitable MACS separator and columns

(9) FITC anti-mouse CD3, APC anti-mouse NK1. 1 (using or labeling mouse NK cells)

(10) Centrifugal tubes, cytometer, pipettes

(11) Super clean bench, CO_2 incubator

(12) Centrifuge, flow cytometry, microscopes

【Procedures】

For human peripheral blood NK cells isolation

1. Isolation of PBMC:

(1) 2 mL of whole blood is drawn into an EDTA anti-coagulation tube.

(2) Add 2 mL PBS into the 15 mL centrifuge tube, and mix well.

(3) Add 4 mL Ficoll-Hypaque to a new centrifugal tube.

(4) Overlay the diluted blood sample onto the Ficoll-Hypaque, ensuring that the blood and Ficoll-Hypaque do not mix.

(5) Centrifuge the cells at 2,000 r /min for 30 min at room temperature. The acceleration is setting at 4, and the deceleration is setting at 2.

(6) After Centrifuge, the blood is divided into some layers, and PBMC is included in the white cloud-like band on the interface of Ficoll-Hypaque (Fig.14 − 1A).

(7) Aspirate the band gently and remove PBMC to another new tube, wash cells with PBS 2 − 3 times at 1,500 r/min for 5 min at room temperature, and discard the supernatant.

(8) Resuspend cell pellet in 1 mL RPMI − 1640, then cells are counted on the cytometer.

2. Negative magnetic selection of NK cells:

(1) Determine PBMC number. Wash PBMC with bead buffer at 1,500 r/min for 5 min at 4℃.

(2) Resuspend cell pellet in 40 μL of buffer per 10^7 total cells.

(3) Add 10 μL of NK Cell Biotin-Antibody Cocktail per 10^7 total cells, mix well and incubate for 5 minutes in the refrigerator (2 − 8℃).

(4) Add 30 μL of buffer per 10^7 total cells.

(5) Add 20 μL of NK Cell MicroBead Cocktail per 10^7 total cells. Mix well and incubate for 10 minutes in the refrigerator (2 − 8℃).

(6) Place MS column in the magnetic field of a suitable MACS Separator (MS column is chosen when the counts of magnetic labeled cells are less than 10^7. LS column is chosen when the counts of magnetic labeled cells are less than 10^8).

(7) Wash the column with appropriate amount of buffer (MS: 500 μL; LS: 3 mL).

(8) Apply cell suspension onto the column. Collect the flow-through fraction.

(9) Repeat (7) twice. The flow-through fraction contains unlabeled cells, representing the enriched NK cells.

(10) Wash the flow-through fraction 2 − 3 times with bead buffer at 1,500 r/min for 5 min at 4℃.

(11) Resuspend cell pellet in 1 mL RPMI − 1640.

(12) Cells are counted on the cytometer. A part of the cells are used the purity detection by flow cytometry.

For mouse spleen NK cells isolation

1. Preparation of splenocytes:

(1) A mouse is sacrificed. Put the mouse into 75% alcohol for 10 minutes. The mice were fixed on the plate in the prone position. Cut and open the skin on the left back. Expose and take out the spleen sterilely and put it in a plate.

(2) Splenocyte suspensions are prepared by passing the spleen through a 40 μm nylon mesh using the flat side of a syringe plunger.

(3) Centrifuge the splenocyte suspension at 1,500 r/min for 5 min at 4℃, discard the supernatant, and resuspend the cell pellet by PBS. Wash the pellet twice with the same centrifuge condition.

(4) For red blood cell lysis, pelleted cells are resuspended in 1 mL ACK buffer per spleen and incubated for 2 min at room temperature.

(5) ACK is quenched with an equal volume of complete medium. Centrifuge at 1 500 r/min for 5 min, discard the supernatant, and collect the cell pellet.

(6) Wash the pellet cells with PBS twice.

(7) Resuspend pellet in 1 mL RPMI-1640. Cells are counted with the cytometer.

2. Negative magnetically selection of NK cells:

(1) Determine splenocyte number. Wash with bead buffer at 1,500 r/min for 5 min at 4℃.

(2) Resuspend cell pellet in 40 μL of buffer per 10^7 total cells.

(3) Add 10 μL of NK Cell Biotin-Antibody Cocktail per 10^7 total cells, mix well and incubate cells for 5 minutes in the refrigerator (2-8℃).

(4) Add 30 μL of buffer per 10^7 total cells.

(5) Add 20 μL of anti-biotin microBead per 10^7 total cells. Mix well and incubate cells for 10 minutes in the refrigerator (2-8℃).

(6) Place LS column in the magnetic field of a suitable MACS Separator (MS column is chosen when the counts of magnetic labeled cells are less than 10^7. LS column is chosen when the counts of magnetic labeled cells are less than 10^8).

(7) Wash the column with appropriate amount of buffer (MS: 500 μL; LS: 3 mL)

(8) Apply cell suspension onto the column. Collect the flow-through fraction.

(9) Repeat (7) twice. The flow-through fraction contains unlabeled cells, representing the enriched NK cells.

(10) Wash the flow-through fraction 2-3 times with bead buffer at 1,500 r/min for 5 min at 4℃.

(11) Resuspend cell pellet in 1 mL RPMI-1640.

(12) Cells are counted on the cytometer. A part of the cells are used for the purity detection by flow cytometry.

【Results】

In this experiment, 70% NK cells can be achieved from PBMC, and the purity of NK cell is more than 85%.

In this experiment, about 65% NK cells can be achieved from the splenic lymphocytes, and the purity of NK cell is more than 85%.

【Precautions】

1. The diluted blood sample should be slowly overlaid onto the Ficoll-Hypaque along the wall of the tube. Do not mix them.

2. It is best to aspirate the white cloud-like band slightly. Try the best to avoid mixing the band with other layer.

3. Keep cells cold, and use pre-cooled buffer $(2-8℃)$.

4. Work fast. Long-time work is prone to make cell death.

5. Do not lyse red blood cells over time, which may cause cell death.

6. A LS column can hold up to 1×10^8 cells; for larger cell quantities, increase the number of LS columns appropriately.

【Questions】

1. What are the benefits of negative selection of NK cells in this protocol?

2. What is the key factor to success in this experiment?

(Gao Ming   Zheng Fang)

实验十五　磁珠分选小鼠脾脏 T 细胞

【原理】

　　免疫磁珠法分离细胞是基于细胞表面抗原能与连接有磁珠的特异性单抗相结合,在外加磁场中,通过抗体与磁珠相连的细胞被吸附而滞留在磁场中,无该种表面抗原的细胞由于不能与连接着磁珠的特异性单抗结合而没有磁性,不在磁场中停留,从而使细胞得以分离。免疫磁珠法分为阴性分选法和阳性分选法。阳性分选法即磁珠结合的细胞就是所要分离获得的细胞;阴性分选法即磁珠结合不需要的细胞,游离于上清液的细胞为所需细胞。一般而言,阴性分选法比阳性分选法的磁珠用量大。免疫学实验中,经常使用阴性分选法来得到所需的免疫细胞。

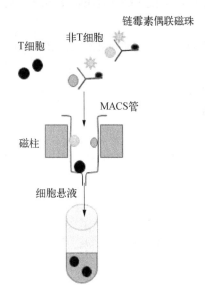

图 15-1　磁珠阴性分选法
分离 T 细胞

非 T 细胞被生物素抗体及链霉素偶联磁珠所标记,非 T 细胞保留在磁柱上,T 细胞流经磁柱后被富集

　　本实验应用阴性分选法来分离小鼠脾脏 T 细胞。首先将单核细胞悬液与小鼠生物素化的抗体悬液一起孵育,该混悬液靶向结合 CD3 阴性细胞。将链霉素蛋白磁珠加到反应体系中,使链霉素偶联磁珠与生物素化的抗体标记的细胞相互作用。然后将含细胞悬液的管子置于磁场中。磁性标记的细胞向磁体(不需要的细胞部分)迁移,使未标记的细胞或所需的细胞群处于悬浮状态,通过抽吸获取,同时管子保留在磁场中。通过这种阴性分选法可获得高纯度的 T 细胞(图 15-1)。

【应用】

　　分离的 T 细胞可用于 T 细胞的功能检测。

【材料】

　　1. 培养液:含 10%牛血清的 Hank's 平衡盐溶液(HBSS)

　　2. 小鼠 $CD3^+T$ 细胞生物素化抗体混悬液

　　3. 链霉素抗生物素蛋白磁珠

　　4. 10×PBS(NaCl 80 g、KCl 2 g、Na_2HPO_4 14.4 g、KH_2PO_4 2.4 g,溶解于 800 mL 蒸馏水,调 pH 至 7.4,补充液体至 1 L。可高压蒸汽灭菌)

　　5. ACK 红细胞裂解液(NH_4CL 8.29 g、$KHCO_3$ 1.00 g、Na_2EDTA 37.2 mg,溶解于 800 mL 蒸馏水,调 pH 至 7.2~7.4,补充液体至 1 L。可高压蒸汽灭菌)

　6. MagCellect 磁铁

　7. 5 mL 或 15 mL 聚苯乙烯管

　8. 无菌巴斯德吸管或移液器

　9. 无菌蒸馏水或去离子水

　10. 40～70 μm 尼龙细胞过滤器

　11. CO_2 培养箱

　12. 层流通风橱

　13. 离心机

【方法】

　1. 分离小鼠脾脏,用含 10% 牛血清的 HBSS 重悬脾脏细胞,细胞悬液通过 40 μm(200目)尼龙细胞过滤器去除细胞团块和/或碎片,制成单细胞悬液。

　2. 将细胞转移至 15 mL 离心管,并将细胞以 1 000 r/min 离心 10 min 洗涤一次。

　3. 倒出上清液,将细胞重悬于加入 5 mL ACK 红细胞的裂解液,充分混匀细胞,室温裂解 5 min。

　4. 1 500 r/min 离心 5 min,弃上清,加入含 10% 牛血清的 10 mL HBSS 培养基洗涤 2次,然后将细胞重悬于 200 μL 冷的 1×PBS 中。

　5. 进行细胞计数,然后用冷的 1×PBS 重悬细胞。将细胞浓度调整为每毫升 $2×10^8$ 个细胞(每 $2×10^8$ 个待处理细胞需用 10 mL 1×PBS)。1×PBS 应保存在冰上或冷藏,并在24 h 内使用。

　6. 将 $2×10^8$ 个细胞(1.0 mL)转移到 5 mL 聚苯乙烯管中,然后加入 200 μL 小鼠 $CD3^+T$ 细胞生物素化抗体混悬液。轻轻混合细胞—抗体悬浮液,避免形成气泡,并在 2～8℃ 的冰箱中孵育 15 min。

　7. 向细胞悬浮液中加入 200 μL 链霉素抗生物素蛋白磁珠,轻轻混合并在 2～8℃ 的冰箱中孵育 15 min。

　8. 在孵育结束时,加入 1.6 mL 1×PBS 缓冲液使管中的反应体积达到 3 mL。轻轻混合以确保管中的所有反应物都处于悬浮状态。

　9. 将反应管放入已水平放置的 MagCellect 磁体中(可容纳 5 mL 试管),并在室温下孵育 6 min。磁性标记的细胞将向磁体迁移(这些是不需要的细胞),使未接触的所需细胞悬浮在上清液中。

　10. 不要取出反应管,使用无菌巴斯德吸管或移液管小心地吸出所有反应上清液并将其置于新的 5 mL 试管中。从磁铁上取下含有磁性捕获细胞的试管,然后丢弃。

　11. 为了确保已除去所有磁珠,用含有回收细胞的新管重复步骤 6 和 7 至磁性耗尽。在这些步骤结束时获得的上清液是含有所需富集的 $CD3^+T$ 细胞的最终部分。

　12. 质量控制:$CD3^+T$ 细胞纯化的程度可通过细胞表面 CD2 和 CD3 抗体标记来测定。

【结果】

　分离得到的 T 细胞纯度经 CD2 和 CD3 抗体检测后,纯度可达 90% 以上。

【注意事项】

1. 如果细胞选择后需要无菌细胞,整个过程应在层流罩中进行,以保持无菌条件。在移液时使用无菌设备。

2. 尽快操作避免非特异性细胞标记,通过使用预冷溶液并遵守方案中指定的孵育时间和温度,使细胞和溶液保持冷却。升高的温度和延长的孵育时间可能导致非特异性细胞标记,从而降低细胞纯度和产量。

3. 处理不同数量的细胞时,保持抗体和磁珠的孵育时间和温度不变;保持细胞密度为 $2×10^8$ 个/mL;每 $1×10^7$ 个细胞加入 10 μL 抗体混合物;每 $1×10^7$ 个细胞加入 10 μL 链霉素抗生物素蛋白磁珠。

【思考题】

磁珠分选分离 T 细胞的原理是什么?

（刘　敏）

Exp. 15　Isolation of T Cell from Mouse Spleen Using Magnetic Beads

【Principle】

Immunomagnetic beads separation of cells is based on the combination of cell surface antigens and specific monoclonal antibodies linked to magnetic beads. In an external magnetic field, cells connected to the magnetic beads by the antibody are adsorbed and retained in the magnetic field. Cells without specific surface antigen are not magnetic due to its inability to bind to a specific monoclonal antibody to which a magnetic bead is attached, and do not stay in a magnetic field, thereby allowing the cells to be separated. The immunomagnetic beads methods are divided into a positive selection method and a negative selection method. For the positive selection method, magnetic beads-bound cells are the cells to be separated; For the negative selection method, magnetic beads combine the unwanted cells, and the cells in the supernatant are the desired cells. In general, the negative selection method uses more amount of magnetic beads than the positive selection method. In immunological experiments, negative selection is often used to obtain the desired immune cells.

In this experiment, negative magnetic selection is used to isolated T cells from mouse spleen. A mononuclear cell suspension is first incubated with the MagCellect Mouse CD3$^+$T Cell Biotinylated Antibody Cocktail which targets the unwanted CD3$^-$T cells. MagCellect Streptavidin Ferrofluid is next added to the reaction and the streptavidin coated beads interact with biotinylated antibody tagged cells. The tube containing the cell suspension is then placed within a magnetic field. Magnetically tagged cells will migrate toward the magnet (unwanted cell fraction), leaving the untagged cells or desired cell population in suspension to be harvested by aspiration while the tube remains in the magnetic field. By this negative magnetic sorting, high purity T cells are obtained (Fig.15 − 1).

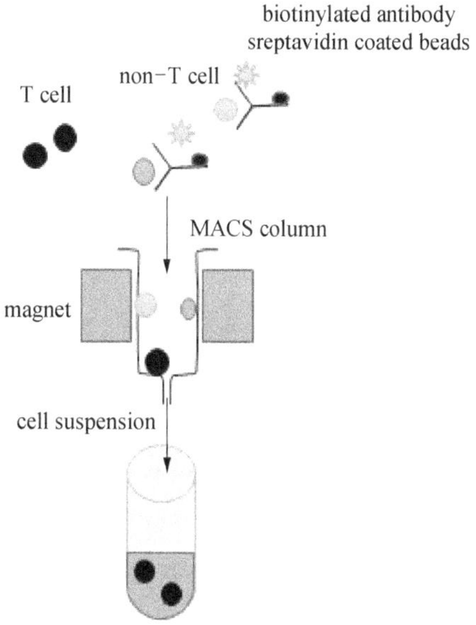

Fig.15 − 1　Isolation of T cell using magnetic beads

Magnetic labelling of non-T cells with biltinylated antibody cocktail and streptavidin coated microbeads. Non-T cells are retained in MACS column placed in a MACS separator. T cells pass through the column and are collected as the enriched, unlabeled cell fraction.

【Application】

Purified T cells can be used for subsequent T cell function testing

【Materials】

1. Culture medium: Hank's balanced salt solution (HBSS) supplemented with 10% bovine serum

2. Mouse CD3$^+$T Cell Biotinylated Antibody Cocktail

3. Streptavidin ferrofluid

4. 10×PBS buffer (80 g NaCl, 2 g KCl, 14.4 g Na$_2$HPO$_4$, 2.4 g KH$_2$PO$_4$, dissolved in 800 mL of distilled water, adjusted to pH 7.4,replenish liquid to 1 L. Autoclaved)

5. ACK lysing buffer (NH$_4$CL 8.29 g, KHCO$_3$ 1.00 g, Na$_2$EDTA 37.2 mg, dissolved in 800 mL distilled water, adjusted the pH to 7.2 – 7.4, replenish the liquid to 1 L. Autoclaved)

6. MagCellect magnet

7. 12 mm×75 mm (5 mL) or 17 mm×100 mm (15 mL) polystyrene round bottom tubes

8. Sterile Pasteur pipettes or transfer pipettes

9. Sterile distilled or deionized water

10. 40 – 70 μm nylon cell strainer

11. CO$_2$ incubator

12. Laminar flow fume hood

13. Centrifuge

【Procedures】

1. Gently tease apart the mouse spleen(s) in order to generate a single cell suspension in Hank's balanced salt solution (HBSS) supplemented with 10% bovine serum. To remove cell clumps and/or debris by passing the suspended cells through a 40 μm (200 mesh)nylon cell strainer.

2. Wash the cells once by filling a 15 mL centrifuge tube and spinning the cells for 10 minutes at 1,000 r/min.

3. Decant the supernatant, resuspend the cells in 5 mL ACK hemocytes, mix well for lysis 5 min at room temperature.

4. Centrifuge at 1,500 r/min for 5 min, discard the supernatant, wash cells twice with 10 mL HBSS medium containing 10% bovine serum, and then resuspend the cells in 200 μL of cold 1×PBS buffer.

5. Perform a cell count and then adjust the cell concentration to 2×10^8 cells per mL with cold 1×PBS Buffer (prepare 10 mL of 1×PBS Buffer for each 2×10^8 cells). The 1× MagCellect Buffer should be kept on ice or refrigerated and used within 24 hours.

6. Transfer 2×10^8 cells (1. 0 mL volume) into a 5 mL polystyrene tube and then add 200 μL of Mouse CD3$^+$T Cell Biotinylated Antibody Cocktail. Gently mix the cell-antibody suspension, avoid bubble formation. Incubate cells at $2-8$℃ in a refrigerator for 15 minutes.

7. Add 200 μL of streptavidin ferrofluid to the cell suspension, mix gently and incubate for 15 min in a refrigerator at $2-8$℃.

8. At the end of the incubation period, bring the volume of the reaction in the tube to 3 mL by adding 1. 6 mL of 1×PBS Buffer. Mix gently to ensure that all reactants in the tube are in suspension.

9. Place the reaction tube in the MagCellect Magnet that has been positioned horizontally (to accommodate 5 mL tubes) and incubate for 6 min at room temperature. Magnetically tagged cells will migrate toward the magnet (these are the unwanted cells), leaving the untouched desired cells in suspension in the supernatant.

10. While the tube is in the magnet, use a sterile Pasteur pipette or transfer pipette to carefully aspirate all of the reaction supernatant and place it in a new 5 mL tube. Remove the tube containing the magnetically trapped cells from the magnet, and discard the tube.

11. To ensure that all of the magnetic nanoparticles have been removed, repeat the magnetic depletion (steps 6 and 7) with the new tube containing the recovered cells. The supernatant obtained at the end of these steps is the final depleted cell fraction containing the desired enriched CD3$^+$T cells.

12. Quality control: The extent of CD3$^+$T cells purification can be determined by cell surface CD2 and CD3 antibody labelled.

【Results】

The purity of T cells obtained from above is tested by CD2 and CD3 antibodies. The purity is up to 90%.

【Precautions】

1. If sterile cells are required following the cell selection, the entire procedure should be carried out in a laminar flow hood to maintain sterile conditions. Use sterile equipment when pipet reagents.

2. Avoid non-specific cell tagging by working fast, keeping cells and solutions by using pre-cooled solutions and following to the incubation times and temperatures specified in the protocol. Increased temperature and prolonged incubation times may lead to non-specific cell labelling thus lowering cell purity and yield.

3. When processing different numbers of cells, keep antibody cocktail and ferrofluid incubation times and temperatures unchanged; keep the cell density at 2×10^8 cells/mL; add 10 μL of the antibody cocktail per 1×10^7 cells being processed; add 10 μL of Streptavidin Ferrofluid per 1×10^7 cells being processed.

【Question】

What is the principle of using magnetic beads for separating T cells?

(Liu Min)

实验十六　尼龙棉法分离小鼠 B 细胞

【原理】

在研究免疫细胞时,常需要先将免疫细胞分离纯化,再进一步进行检测。通常可根据细胞的表面标志、理化性质及功能进行设计和选择不同的分离方法对所需细胞进行纯化分离。

混合细胞悬液在通过尼龙棉柱时,B 细胞易黏附于尼龙棉纤维表面,而 T 细胞不易黏附并随液体流出,由此达到分离 B 细胞的目的。

【应用】

分离纯化 B 细胞。用于 B 细胞功能分析。

【材料】

1. RPMI – 1640 培养液
2. 10% FBS – RPMI – 1640 培养液
3. 0.2 mol/L HCl 溶液
4. Hank's 液(NaCl 0.137 mol/L, KCl 5.4 mmol/L, Na_2HPO_4 0.25 mmol/L, 葡萄糖 0.1 g, KH_2PO_4 0.44 mmol/L, 1.3 mmol/L $CaCl_2$, 1.0 mmol/L $MgSO_4$, 4.2 mmol/L $NaHCO_3$, 可高压蒸汽灭菌)
5. ACK 红细胞裂解液(NH_4Cl 8.29 g、$KHCO_3$ 1.00 g、Na_2EDTA 37.2 mg,溶解于 800 mL 蒸馏水,调 pH 至 7.2~7.4,补充水至 1 L。可高压蒸汽灭菌)
6. 塑料软管(0.5 cm, 15 cm)
7. 尼龙棉
8. 玻璃平皿、玻璃试管和玻璃吸管
9. 超净工作台和 CO_2 孵箱

【方法】

1. 小鼠脾细胞获取
(1) 颈椎脱臼处死小鼠,75% 乙醇浸泡 10 min。
(2) 无菌条件下取出小鼠脾脏,将其放置于盛有 4℃ 预冷 RPMI – 1640 培养基的 60 mm 培养皿中,放入钢丝滤网,用注射器头研磨,至未见明显脾脏组织团块。
(3) 将脾脏细胞悬液收集至 15 mL 离心管中,1 500 r/min 离心 5 min,弃上清。
(4) 加入 5 mL ACK 红细胞裂解液,室温裂解 5 min。
(5) 1 500 r/min 离心 5 min,弃上清,加入 10 mL RPMI – 1640 培养液洗涤 2 次后,用 10% FBS – RPMI – 1640 培养液重悬细胞,用于后续实验。

2. 准备尼龙棉柱

(1) 将 0.2 g 尼龙棉撕匀,0.2 mol/L HCl 浸泡 24 h。

(2) 尼龙棉用大量蒸馏水冲洗后,平铺于玻璃皿,50℃干燥箱内烘干(12 h)。

(3) 尼龙棉高压灭菌。

(4) 酒精洗手两遍,在超净台内撕匀尼龙棉,用细棍将尼龙棉引入玻璃吸管中部,两端空出 2 cm。

(5) 用 Hank's 液反复冲洗,最后一次用预温至 37℃的 10% FBS‐RPMI‐1640 培养液洗柱。

3. 尼龙棉柱分离 B 细胞

(1) 调整淋巴细胞数至 2×10^7/mL,吸取 0.5 mL 垂直加入尼龙棉柱,平放尼龙棉柱,以细长的滴管伸入柱内近尼龙棉界面,滴加适量的 10% FBS‐RPMI‐1640 培养液,以免尼龙棉干燥。

(2) 将棉柱平放于 37℃温箱中孵育 30 min。

(3) 柱子垂直放入 10 mL 玻璃试管,注射器吸取 5~10 mL 37℃预温的 10% FBS‐RPMI‐1640 缓缓注入柱子(约 60 滴/min),此时收集的洗脱液富含 T 细胞。

(4) 柱子放于第二支玻璃试管中,注射器吸取 20~25 mL 37℃预热的 10% FBS‐RPMI‐1640 培养液,以同样方式洗涤,以充分洗去残余 T 细胞。

(5) 尼龙棉柱放入第三支玻璃管,注射器吸取 5 mL 冰冷的 10% FBS‐RPMI‐1640 培养液,缓缓注入尼龙棉柱并从上往下轻轻挤压柱子,此时收集的洗脱液中富含 B 细胞(冰冷的 10% FBS‐RPMI‐1640 培养液可降低 B 细胞的黏附性,通过挤压利于 B 细胞被洗脱下来)。

【结果】

通过此法成功收集到 B 细胞,可用流式细胞术检测其 CD19+ B 细胞的纯度。

【注意事项】

1. 该方法所需实验材料简单,操作简便,但获得的 B 细胞纯度不高。

2. 制备好的尼龙棉柱在冲洗和过柱分离时,要保证没有气泡产生,否则会影响分离效果。

3. 将淋巴细胞悬液加入尼龙棉柱后,要立即补加 37℃预温的 10% FBS‐RPMI‐1640 培养液,以防尼龙棉干燥影响淋巴细胞活性。

【思考题】

简述尼龙棉柱分离 B 细胞的原理。

(潘　勤)

Exp. 16　Isolation and Purification of B Cells by Nylon Wool

【Principle】

The specific population of immune cells usually need isolation and purification from heterogeneous cell pool for phenotypic and functional analysis. These specific population of immune cells can be isolated and purified according to the surface markers, physical and chemical properties and functions.

When the immune cells are filtered through nylon wool column, the B cells adhere to nylon wool, whereas the T cells do not adhere and then they can be eluted from the column.

【Application】

Isolation and purification of B cells. B cell functional analysis.

【Materials】

1. RPMI－1640 medium
2. 10% FBS－RPMI－1640 medium
3. 0.2 mol/L HCl solution
4. Hank's solution (NaCl 0.137 mol/L, KCl 5.4 mmol/L, Na_2HPO_4 0.25 mmol/L, glucose 0.1 g, KH_2PO_4 0.44 mmol/L, $CaCl_2$ 1.3 mmol/L, $MgSO_4$ 1.0 mmol/L, $NaHCO_3$ 4.2 mmol/L, autoclaved)
5. ACK lysing buffer (NH_4Cl 8.29 g, $KHCO_3$ 1.00 g, Na_2EDTA 37.2 mg, dissolved in 800 mL distilled water, adjusted the pH to 7.2－7.4, replenish the H_2O to 1 L, autoclaved)
6. Plastic hose (0.5 cm, 15 cm)
7. Nylon wool
8. Glass plate, glass tube and glass straw
9. Ultra-clean fume hood, CO_2 incubator

【Procedures】

1. Murine spleen cell preparation:

(1) Mice are sacrificed by cervical dislocation and soaked in 75% alcohol for 10 min.

(2) The mouse spleen is removed under aseptic conditions, and placed in 4℃ pre-cooling RPMI－1640 medium in a 60 mm cell culture dish. The spleen tissue is homogenized by using the plunger end of a syringe on a wire mesh until no visible fragments are observed.

(3) Collect the cells in 15 mL centrifuge tubes. Centrifuge the cell suspension at 1 500 r/min

for 5 min, and discard the supernatant.

(4) Resuspend the cell pellets in 5 mL ACK buffer. Incubate for 5 min at room temperature.

(5) Centrifuge at 1 500 r/min for 5 min at room temperature and remove the supernatant carefully. After washed with 10 mL of RPMI – 1640 for 2 times, cells are filtered through a nylon mesh filter to further remove connective tissues and other debris.

(6) Resuspend the cell pellets in 10% FBS – RPMI – 1640 medium.

2. Prepare nylon wool column:

(1) 0.2 g of nylon wool is soaked in 0.2 mol/L HCl for 24 h.

(2) After rinsed with distilled H_2O, nylon wool is placed on a glass dish and dried at 50℃ for 12 h.

(3) Autoclave the nylon wool.

(4) Wash your hands twice with alcohol, tear the nylon wool into small pieces in the ultra-clean fume hood. Stuff the nylon wool into the middle of the glass straw with a thin stick, and leave 2 cm at both ends of the straw.

(5) Rinse the nylon wool with Hank's solution repeatedly, and wash the column with 10% FBS – RPMI – 1640 medium at the last rinse.

3. Isolation and purification of B cells by nylon wool column:

(1) Vertically add 0.5 mL of cell suspension ($2×10^7$/mL) to the nylon wool column. Convert the nylon wool column to the horizontal position. Add small amount of 10% FBS – RPMI – 1640 medium to avoid nylon wool be dried.

(2) Incubate the column in a 37℃ incubator for 30 min.

(3) The column is vertically placed into a 10 mL glass tube, and 5 – 10 mL of 10% FBS – RPMI – 1640 medium is slowly added into the column (about 60 drops/min) by the syringe. At this time, the eluted cells are rich in T cells.

(4) The column is placed in another glass tube, and 20 – 25 mL of 10% FBS – RPMI – 1640 medium are employed in rinse to elute the residual T cells.

(5) Put the column into the third glass tube, slowly add 5 mL of ice-cold 10% FBS – RPMI – 1640 medium into the column, and gently squeeze the column from top to bottom. Collected B cells are enriched in the eluted cell suspension. (Icy RPMI – 1640+10% FBS can reduce the adhesion of B cells, which is beneficial for B cells to be eluted).

【Results】

B cells were collected by this method. The percentages of B cells in collected cell suspension can be determined by flow cytometry.

【Precautions】

1. The method for isolation and purification of B cells by nylon wool is simple and easy

to be operated, but the purity of collected B cells is not high.

2. Ensure no bubble in the prepared nylon wool column when rinsing the column, otherwise the bubble will hinder the isolation.

3. After adding the cell suspension into the column, immediately add 10% FBS –RPMI – 1640 medium to prevent nylon wool be dried, otherwise cell activity will be reduced during the isolation.

【Question】

Describe the principle of B cells isolation by nylon wool column.

(Pan Qin)

实验十七　磁珠分选 B 细胞

【原理】

表达特定表面分子的细胞能与连接有磁珠的相应单抗特异性结合。在外加磁场中，被磁珠标记的细胞被滞留在磁场中，无特定表面分子的细胞，由于不能与磁珠连接，不受磁场的影响。这些细胞不在磁场中停留，会随着液体流出。通过以上原理，使携带有不同表面标记抗原的细胞得以分离(图 17-1)。

本实验介绍的是阴性分选法从小鼠的脾细胞中分离纯化 B 细胞。

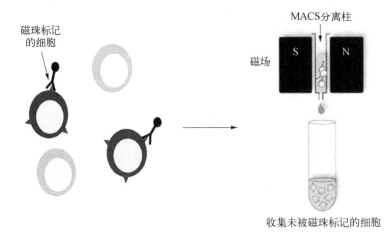

图 17-1　磁珠分选 B 细胞(阴性分选法)

【应用】

B 细胞的分离纯化，B 细胞功能检测。

【材料】

1. 缓冲液：PBS(pH 7.2)中含有 0.5% BSA 和 2 mmol/L EDTA
2. 小鼠生物素标记抗体(混合抗体)：包括生物素标记的抗 CD43、CD4 和 Ter-119 单克隆抗体
3. 抗生物素抗体偶联的磁珠
4. MACS 分离柱
5. 脾细胞悬液

【方法】

1. 小鼠脾细胞获取：同实验十六。

2. 磁珠分离 B 细胞：

（1）准备小鼠脾细胞,确定细胞浓度。

（2）每 $1×10^7$ 个细胞用 40 μL PBS 重悬细胞。

（3）每 $1×10^7$ 个细胞加 10 μL 链霉素标记的抗体。

（4）将抗体与细胞混匀并放入 4℃冰箱 5 min。

（5）每 $1×10^7$ 个细胞中加 30 μL PBS。

（6）每 $1×10^7$ 个细胞悬液中加 20 μL 生物素标记的磁珠。

（7）充分混匀,并置 4℃冰箱中孵育 10 min。

（8）取出分离柱子放在架子上置于磁场中,柱子下方放置 15 mL 离心管。

（9）加细胞悬液到分离柱中,再加 3 mL PBS 冲洗柱子。

（10）收集滤过分离柱的细胞,即为所需的 B 细胞。

【结果】

通过此法成功收集到 B 细胞,可用流式细胞术检测 B 细胞的纯度。

【注意事项】

1. 如果细胞分选后需要无菌培养细胞,整个分选过程应在无菌条件下进行。

2. 操作时应注意预冷和细胞的低温保持。温度的升高和孵育时间的延长可能导致非特异性细胞标记,从而降低细胞纯度和产量。

【思考题】

为什么一般都用磁珠阴性分选方法进行免疫细胞的纯化和功能检测?

（潘　勤）

Exp. 17 Isolation and Purification of B Cells by MACS

【Principle】

The method of immunomagnetic beads separation is based on the binding ability of cells which express corresponding surface markers with specific monoclonal antibodies linked to magnetic beads. In an external magnetic field, the immunomagnetic beads carrying the corresponding cells are adsorbed and retained in the magnetic field. The cells without surface antigen are not magnetic due to their inability of binding with the specific monoclonal antibody to which the magnetic beads are attached, and do not stay in the magnetic field, and thereby the cells can be separated (Fig.17 − 1).

In the present experiment, the murine splenic B cells will be isolated and purified by negative selection.

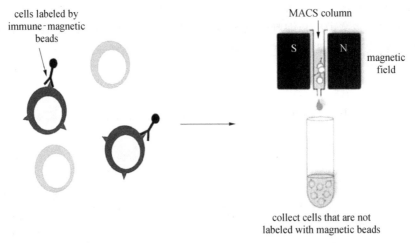

cells labeled by immune-magnetic beads

MACS column

magnetic field

collect cells that are not labeled with magnetic beads

Fig.17 − 1   B cell isolation and purification by MACS (negative selection)

【Application】

Isolation and purification of B cells. B cell functional analysis.

【Materials】

1. Buffer: prepare a solution containing phosphate-buffered saline (PBS), pH 7.2, 0.5% bovine serum albumin (BSA), and 2 mmol/L EDTA

2. Mouse biotin-antibody cocktail: cocktail of biotin-conjugated monoclonal antibodies against CD43, CD4, and Ter-119

3. Microbeads conjugated to monoclonal anti-biotin antibodies

4. MACS column

5. Splenocyte suspension

[Procedures]

1. Murine spleen cell preparation (see Exp.16).

2. B cell isolation:

(1) Prepare mouse splenocytes and count cell number.

(2) Resuspend cell pellets in 40 μL of buffer per 10^7 total cells.

(3) Add 10 μL of biotin-antibody cocktail per 10^7 total cells.

(4) Mix well and incubate in the refrigerator at 4℃ for 5 min.

(5) Add 30 μL of PBS buffer per 10^7 total cells.

(6) Add 20 μL of anti-biotin microbeads per 10^7 total cells.

(7) Mix well and incubate in the refrigerator at 4℃ for 10 min.

(8) Place column in the magnetic field of a suitable MACS separator, and place 15 mL centrifuge tube under the column.

(9) Apply cell suspension into the column, add 3 mL of PBS buffer and continue to wash the remaining cells.

(10) Collect flow-through containing unlabelled cells which representing the enriched B cells.

[Results]

B cells were successfully collected by this method. The percentage of B cells can be determined by flow cytometry.

[Precautions]

1. If cells are required to be cultured after MACS isolation, the entire procedure should be carried out in a laminar flow hood to maintain aseptic conditions.

2. Keep cells and solutions cold by using pre-cooled solutions. Increased temperature and prolonged incubation times may lead to non-specific cell labelling thus reducing cell purity and yield.

[Question]

Why is negative selection usually used in MACS isolation for cell functional analysis?

(Pan Qin)

实验十八　小鼠肺泡巨噬细胞的分离和纯化

【原理】

肺泡巨噬细胞存在于肺泡组织中。肺泡巨噬细胞的生物活性较高,它们在气道、支气管和肺泡中清除灰尘或微生物等颗粒。本实验介绍通过支气管肺泡灌洗术从小鼠肺组织中分离和纯化肺泡巨噬细胞。

【应用】

分离和纯化肺泡巨噬细胞,供体外检测巨噬细胞数量和功能。

【材料】

1. PBS－EDTA 溶液:不含 Mg 离子和 Ca 离子,含 0.6 mmol/L EDTA 的 PBS,无菌
2. 台盼蓝溶液
3. 10% FBS－RPMI－1640 培养液
4. SURFLO I.V. 导管 18Gx1 ¼ (Terumo,Ref. SR－OX1832CF)
5. 1 mL 注射器
6. 50 mL 离心管,无菌
7. 六孔板

【方法】

1. 处死小鼠。用 75% 乙醇浸湿小鼠表面皮毛。使用剪刀在小鼠颈部皮肤上做一个小切口,露出颈部(图 18－1)。
2. 手术操作暴露气管。
3. 使用 SURFLO 导管进行气管插管。在进行灌洗时,将一只手放在导管上,并用钳子稳定气管,或使用缝线将气管和导管接口处固定。
4. 用 1 mL 注射器吸取 0.5 mL 无菌冰冷的无 Mg 离子和 Ca 离子的 PBS－EDTA。
5. 将注射器放在 SURFLO 导管的末端,通过导管小心地将盐水注入动物肺部。
6. 拉动注射器针管,将肺部灌洗液吸出。
7. 从导管中取出注射器,将灌洗液收集到 50 mL 离心管(置于冰上)中。
8. 重复步骤:用 1 mL PBS－EDTA 灌洗肺部 4~8 次。
9. 将收集的灌洗液置冰上,定容至 10 mL 并充分混合。
10. 将 10 μL 灌洗液与 10 μL 台盼蓝混合。通过光学显微镜计数活细胞。
11. 将剩余的灌洗液以 1 500 r/min 离心 10 min,并弃去上清液。
12. 如果后续进行流式细胞术检测,将细胞沉淀重悬于冷 PBS 中进行检测。
13. 如果后续进行细胞培养,将细胞重悬在温热的 10% FBS－RPMI－1640 培养液

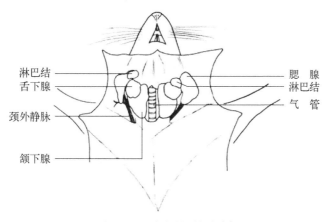

图 18 - 1 小鼠的颈部解剖

中,并使细胞浓度达到 2×10^6 个 /mL,每孔 2 mL 细胞悬液,在六孔板中培养。细胞放入 37℃ 培养箱中 45 min,使巨噬细胞黏附贴壁。

【结果】

用此法收集肺泡巨噬细胞。通过台盼蓝染色和光学显微镜观察细胞活力。收集的肺泡巨噬细胞的占比可通过流式细胞术确定。

【注意事项】

1. 使用注射器时要特别小心,勿让针头刺穿导管。

2. 使用该方法可以收集到大约 50% 的肺泡巨噬细胞,肺泡至少要灌洗 5 次。

3. 在含有 5% CO_2 的 37℃ 培养箱中培养巨噬细胞,在血清存在的条件下,巨噬细胞牢固地黏附于培养板孔上。

【思考题】

巨噬细胞在参与机体免疫应答中有哪些生物学功能?

(潘 勤)

Exp. 18 Isolation and Purification of Murine Alveolar Macrophages

【Principle】

An alveolar macrophage is a type of macrophage found in the pulmonary alveolus. The activities of the alveolar macrophage are relatively high, and they are responsible for removing particles such as dust or microorganisms from the respiratory surfaces. The current experiment describes isolation and purification of murine alveolar macrophages from the lungs by bronchoalveolar lavage (BAL).

【Application】

Isolation and purification of alveolar macrophages. Functional analysis of alveolar macrophages.

【Materials】

1. Mg^{2+}-and Ca^{2+}-free PBS +0. 6 mmol/L EDTA (PBS－EDTA), sterile
2. Trypan blue solution
3. 10% FBS－RPMI－1640 medium
4. SURFLO I. V. catheter 18G×1 ¼ (Terumo, Ref. SR－OX1832CF)
5. 1 mL syringe
6. 50 mL tube, sterile
7. 6-well tissue culture plate

【Procedures】

1. The mice are sacrificed. Dampen the mouse fur with 75% ethanol. Using scissors make a small incision in the animal skin at the neck. Peal skin upwards to expose the neck (Fig.18－1).

2. Dissect tissue from neck to expose trachea.

3. Cannulate the trachea using a SURFLO catheter. Keep one hand on the catheter while proceeding with the lavages. Stabilize trachea with forceps throughout the procedure or tie the trachea around the catheter using sutures.

4. Load a 1 mL syringe with 0. 5 mL sterile ice-cold Mg^{2+}-and Ca^{2+}-free PBS－EDTA.

5. Place syringe in the end of the SURFLO catheter. Carefully inject saline into the animal lungs.

6. Aspirate saline by pulling barrel of syringe.

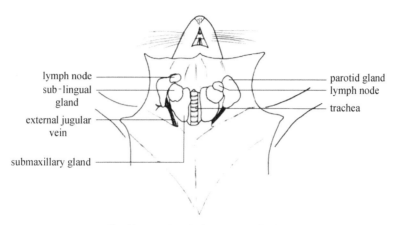

Fig.18 − 1   Cervical anatomy of mice

7. Remove syringe from the catheter, eject recovered lavage fluid into 50 mL tube on ice.

8. Repeat procedure: wash with 1 mL PBS − EDTA 4 − 8 times.

9. Pool lavages on ice. Add PBS − EDTA to 10 mL and mix them well.

10. Mix 10 μL of lavage fluid with 10 μL Trypan blue. Count viable cells by light microscopy.

11. Centrifuge remaining lavage at 1 500 r/min for 10 min and discard supernatant.

12. For flow cytometry, resuspend cell pellet in cold PBS.

13. For cultivation, resuspend in warm 10% FBS − RPMI − 1640 medium and bring cell concentration to 2×10^6 cells/mL. Aliquot 2 mL per well into a 6-well plate. Place into incubator for 45 minutes to allow macrophages to adhere.

【Results】

Alveolar macrophages are collected by this method. The cell viability can be observed by trypan blue staining and light microscopy. The percentages of alveolar macrophages in collected cell suspension can be determined by flow cytometry.

【Precautions】

1. Use special caution with syringe needles and refer to the proper disposal procedure for sharps.

2. Up to circa 50% of total alveolar macrophages can be retrieved using this protocol. A minimum of 5 times are required to flush out most of alveolar macrophages.

3. Cultivate macrophages in a humidified incubator at 37℃ containing 5% humidified CO_2. Macrophages adhere firmly to plate well when cultivated on tissue culture plastic (TCP) or bacteriological plastic (BP) in the presence of serum.

【Question】

What are the biological functions of macrophages involved in the immune function?

(Pan Qin)

实验十九　　小鼠肠道免疫细胞获取

【原理】

肠道免疫系统通过对食物抗原和共生菌产生免疫耐受,而对肠道致病微生物产生有效的免疫应答,在维持胃肠道屏障功能方面发挥重要作用。此外,已经明确肠道局部免疫对远程和系统性免疫有深远的影响。肠道免疫系统的免疫细胞由派尔集合淋巴结(PP)、引流肠系膜淋巴结(MLN)、固有层(LP)和肠上皮(IE)间的免疫细胞组成(图19-1)。

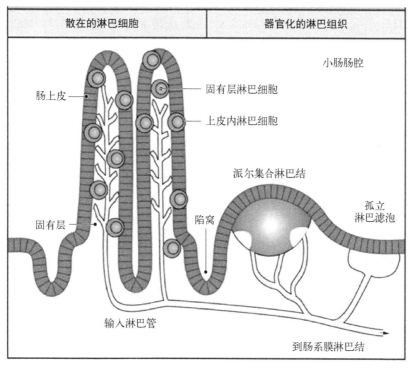

图 19-1　肠道相关的淋巴组织

【应用】

从肠组织中分离免疫细胞有助于研究胃肠道感染、癌症和炎性疾病的免疫应答。

【材料】

1. 剪刀,弯剪,镊子,巴斯德吸管,50 mL 锥形管,15 mL 锥形管,14 mL 聚丙烯圆底管,70 μm 细胞滤器,3 mL 注射器
2. 70%乙醇
3. 离心机,摇床

4. 溶液准备:

(1) HGPG,100×:混合 59.6 g HEPES(500 mmol/L)、14.6 g L-谷氨酰胺(200 mmol/L)、$1×10^6$ U 青霉素(2 000 U/mL)、1 g 链霉素(2 mg/mL)和 2.5 mg 庆大霉素(5 μg/mL),加入 RPMI-1640 至 500 mL。用 NaOH 将 pH 调节至 7.5(调节之前缓冲液为黄色/橙色,pH 约为 6.0)。用 0.45 μm 滤器过滤灭菌,分装并在 -20℃ 下储存长达 1 年或在 4℃ 下储存长达 1 个月。

(2) HEPES-碳酸氢盐缓冲液,10×:混合 23.8 g HEPES(100 mmol/L)、21 g NaHCO₃(250 mmol/L),加水至 1 000 mL。用 HCl 调节 pH 至 7.2。用 0.45 μm 滤器过滤灭菌,室温下储存。pH 随时间变化,定期重新调整。

(3) 培养液:向 500 mL RPMI-1640 中加入 25 mL 热灭活的胎牛血清(5%)和 5 mL 100×HGPG,4℃ 下储存长达 6 个月。

(4) DTE 溶液:50 mL 10×Hank's 平衡盐溶液(不含 Ca^{2+} 和 Mg^{2+})、50 mL 10×HEPES-碳酸氢盐缓冲液和 50 mL 热灭活的胎牛血清(10%)混合,加入 350 mL H_2O 和 15.4 mg DTE/100 mL(1 mmol/L)。使用前新鲜配制。

(5) 乙二胺四乙酸(EDTA)溶液:将 50 mL 10×Hank's 平衡盐溶液(不含 Ca^{2+} 和 Mg^{2+})与 5 mL 100×HGPG 混合,加入 445 mL H_2O。加入 260 μL 0.5 mol/L EDTA/100 mL(1.3 mmol/L)。使用前新鲜配制。

(6) 胶原酶溶液:向 500 mL RPMI 中加入 50 mL FBS(10%)、5 mL 100×HPGP、1 mL 0.5 mol/L $MgCl_2$(终浓度 1 mmol/L)和 1 mL 0.5 mol/L $CaCl_2$(终浓度 1 mmol/L)。加入 I 型胶原酶(100 U/mL)。使用前新鲜配制。

(7) 密度梯度(DG)溶液:① 将 90 mL DG 储备溶液与 10 mL 10×PBS 混合,制备 1×DG 储备溶液。4℃ 无菌保存。② 混合 44 mL 1×DG 储备溶液和 56 mL RPMI-1640,制备 44% DG 溶液。使用前新鲜配制。③ 混合 67 mL 1×DG 储备液和 33 mL RPMI-1640,制备 67% DG 溶液。使用前新鲜配制。

【步骤】

1. 获取肠系膜淋巴结,肠和 Peyer's 淋巴结:

(1) 颈椎脱位法处死小鼠,70% 乙醇消毒。用剪刀做中线切口,打开皮肤和腹壁,露出腹腔。

(2) 轻轻取下 MLN 链在滤纸上滚动去除肠系膜/脂肪,并用两套镊子去掉脂肪,将 MLN 置于培养基中以备在后续分离步骤中使用。

(3) 切开小肠,放在用培养液润湿的纸巾上,用镊子去掉剩余的肠系膜/脂肪。

(4) 用弯剪将派尔集合淋巴结从肠道中取出,放入冷培养基中,以备在后续分离步骤中使用。

(5) 使用镊子的扁平侧,从十二指肠轻轻滑向回肠,排出粪便和黏液。重复一次以去除大部分黏液。

(6) 切开肠道,从十二指肠到回肠纵向打开,横向切成 2 cm 的小块置于 50 mL 锥形管中,加入 25 mL 冷培养基用于后续分离步骤。

2. 从 MLN 和 PP 中分离免疫细胞:

（1）用 70 μm 细胞滤器轻柔地分离 MLN 细胞,并用 5 mL 培养液洗涤细胞滤器。

（2）4℃、1 500 r/min 离心 5 min,1 mL 培养液重悬细胞沉淀。

（3）将派尔集合淋巴结置于含有 5 mL 预热胶原酶溶液的 15 mL 锥形管中,37℃、220 r/min 在摇床上孵育 30 min。

（4）用 70 μm 细胞滤器过滤消化的组织和上清液于 50 mL 锥形管中。用 3 mL 注射器的柱塞轻轻研磨剩余的组织块,并用 5 mL 培养液洗涤细胞滤器。

（4）4℃、1 500 r/min 离心 5 min,并将细胞沉淀重悬于 1 mL 培养基中。

3. 从肠道中分离上皮内免疫细胞:

（1）25 mL 培养基洗涤小肠片 3 次,使肠片沉淀,倒出上清液。

（2）向含有肠片的 50 mL 锥形管中加入 20 mL 预热的 DTE 溶液（DTE 是一种富集上皮内淋巴细胞的还原剂）,并转移至 50 mL 硅化锥形瓶中。37℃、220 r/min 摇 20 min,然后将组织和溶液转移回 50 mL 锥形管。

（3）将管子在最大设置下涡旋 10 s。用 70 μm 细胞滤器将上清液转移到新的 50 mL 锥形管中,小心地将组织碎片保留在原始管中。不要丢弃上清液,上清液含有上皮内淋巴细胞,4℃、1 500 r/min 离心 5 min,将细胞沉淀重悬于 10 mL 冷培养液中,冰上储存。

（4）重复步骤（2）和（3）。将上清液通过 70 μm 细胞滤器转移到第一次 DTE 处理的上清液中。

（5）4℃、1 500 r/min 离心上清液 5 min。室温下将细胞沉淀重悬于 8 mL 44% DG 溶液中。

（6）将 8 mL 44% DG 溶液/细胞悬浮液转移到 14 mL 聚丙烯圆底管中。用 5 mL RT 67% DG 溶液铺底,室温下 5 000 r/min 离心 20 min。

（7）活细胞在 44%至 67%界面处形成条带（棕黄层）,死细胞和一些上皮细胞位于顶部的黏液膜中,红细胞处于沉淀中。将上层吸弃至界面 2 cm 以内,再用巴斯德吸管在界面处收集棕黄层并将其转移至含有 40 mL 冷培养液的 50 mL 锥形管中。

（8）4℃、1 500 r/min 离心 5 min,将细胞沉淀重悬于 1 mL 培养基中。

4. 从小肠中分离固有层免疫细胞:

（1）加入 25 mL 预热的 EDTA 溶液（EDTA 是钙螯合剂,靶向钙依赖性连接并促进肠上皮细胞脱离）至含有剩余肠道的烧瓶中,以去除肠组织碎片中的上皮细胞。37℃、220 r/min 摇 30 min,小心地丢弃上清液,将肠块保持在烧瓶内。

（2）重复上一步骤。

（3）向烧瓶中加入 50 mL RT 培养基。使肠块沉淀并小心地丢弃上清液。

（4）加入 30 mL 预热的胶原酶溶液,37℃、220 r/min 摇 45 min。

（5）通过 70 μm 细胞滤器过滤,将消化的组织和上清液转移到 50 mL 锥形管中。用 3 mL 注射器的柱塞轻轻研磨剩余的组织碎片通过滤器与其混合。用 10 mL 冷培养液清洗过滤器。

（6）4℃、1 500 r/min 离心 5 min,将细胞沉淀重悬于 8 mL 常温的 44% DG 溶液中。

（7）将 8 mL 44% DG 溶液/细胞悬浮液转移到 14 mL 聚丙烯圆底管中。用 5 mL 常温的 67% DG 溶液铺底,25℃ 5 000 r/min 离心 20 min。

(8) 去除顶部的脂肪层,使用巴斯德吸管在界面处收集棕黄层并转移至含有 40 mL 培养基的 50 mL 锥形管中。

(9) 4℃、1 500 r/min 离心 5 min,将细胞沉淀重悬于 1 mL 冷培养基中。

【结果】

可获得高产量、高纯度、高活力的淋巴细胞和固有免疫细胞,如树突细胞、巨噬细胞、中性粒细胞和单核细胞。分离的免疫细胞可以进行进一步的操作,如流式细胞分析或功能分析。

【注意事项】

1. 尽可能多地去除肠道的肠系膜/脂肪以获得最佳的细胞产量和活力。

2. 黏液去除不完全会降低细胞活力和产量。一定要轻轻滑动肠道以避免剥离绒毛或损坏基底膜。

3. 如果出血,可用红细胞裂解液去除红细胞。

【思考题】

1. DTE 和 EDTA 的作用是什么?

2. 在这个实验中必须注意什么?

(史君宇   郑   芳)

Exp. 19   Isolation of Immune Cells from the Mouse Intestinal Immune System

【Principle】

The intestinal immune system plays an essential role in maintaining the barrier function of the gastrointestinal tract by generating tolerant responses to dietary antigens and commensal bacteria while mounting effective immune responses to enteropathogenic microbes. In addition, it has become clear that local intestinal immunity has a profound impact on distant and systemic immunity. The intestinal immune system consists of immune cells from Peyer's patches (PP), draining mesenteric lymph nodes (MLN), lamina propria (LP) and intestinal epithelium (IE) (Fig.19 − 1).

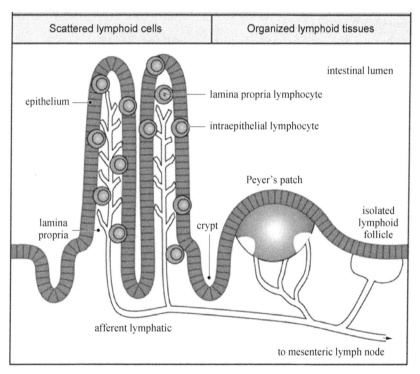

Fig 19 − 1   Gut associated lymphoid tissue

【Application】

The isolation of immune cells from intestinal tissues enables the understanding of immune responses to gastrointestinal infections, cancers, and inflammatory diseases.

【Materials】

1. Scissors, curved scissors, forceps, Pasteur pipette, 50 mL conical tube, 15 mL conical tube, 14 mL polypropylene round-bottom tube, 70 μm cell strainer, 3 mL syringe

2. 70% ethanol

3. Centrifugal, orbital shaker

4. Solution Preparation:

(1) HGPG, 100×: mix 59.6 g HEPES (500 mmol/L final), 14.6 g L-glutamine (200 mmol/L final), 1×10^6 U penicillin (2,000 U/mL final), 1 g streptomycin (2 mg/mL final), and 2.5 mg gentamicin (5 μg/mL final). Add RPMI－1640 medium to 500 mL. Adjust pH to 7.5 using NaOH (before adjustment, the buffer is yellow/orange with a pH around 6.0). Filter sterilize using a 0.45 μm filter. Aliquot and store at -20℃ for up to 1 year or at 4℃ for up to 1 month.

(2) HEPES-bicarbonate buffer, 10×: mix 23.8 g HEPES (100 mmol/L final), 21 g $NaHCO_3$ (250 mmol/L final) and add water to 1,000 mL. Adjust pH to 7.2 with HCl. Filter sterilize using a 0.45 μm filter. Store at room temperature. The pH changes over time. Re-adjust pH periodically.

(3) Media: to 500 mL RPMI－1640 by adding 25 mL heat-inactivated fetal bovine serum (5% final), and 5 mL 100×HGPG. Store up to 6 months at 4℃.

(4) Dithioerythritol (DTE) solution: mix 50 mL 10× Hank's balanced salt solution, Ca^{2+} and Mg^{2+} free, 50 mL 10× HEPES-bicarbonate buffer, and 50 mL heat-inactivated fetal bovine serum (10% final). Add 350 mL H_2O and 15.4 mg DTE/100 mL (1 mmol/L final). Freshly prepare this before use.

(5) Ethylenediaminetetraacetic acid (EDTA) solution: mix 50 mL 10×Hank's balanced salt solution, Ca^{2+}-and Mg^{2+}-free with 5 mL 100×HGPG. Add 445 mL H_2O. Add 260 μL 0.5 mol/L EDTA/100 mL (1.3 mmol/L final). Prepare this fresh before use.

(6) Collagenase solution (30 mL/LP): to 500 mL RPMI, add 50 mL FBS (10% FBS final), 5 mL 100×HPGP, 1 mL 0.5 mol/L $MgCl_2$ (1 mmol/L final), and 1 mL 0.5 mol/L $CaCl_2$ (1 mmol/L final). Add collagenase, Type I (100 U/mL final). Freshly prepare this before use.

(7) Density gradient (DG) solutions: ① Prepare 1×DG stock solution by mixing 90 mL DG stock solution (refer to the Table of Materials) with 10 mL of 10×PBS. Keep sterile at 4℃. ② Prepare 44% DG solution (8 mL/IEL, 8 mL/LP) by mixing 44 mL of 1×DG stock solution and 56 mL RPMI－1640. Freshly prepare this before use.

③ Prepare 67% DG solution (5 mL/IEL, 5 mL/LP) by mixing 67 mL of 1×DG stock solution and 33 mL RPMI－1640. Freshly prepare this before use.

【Procedures】

1. Isolation of the mesenteric lymph nodes, intestines, and Peyer's patches:

(1) The mouse is sacrificed using cervical dislocation and sterilized with 70% ethanol.

Use scissors to make a midline incision, and open the skin and abdominal wall to expose the peritoneal cavity.

（2）Gently remove the MLN chain and remove mesentery/fat by rolling the chain on the paper tower and pulling the fat off with two sets of forceps. And then place the MLN in cold harvest media for later isolation steps.

（3）Cut the small intestine and place the intestine on a paper towel moistened with harvest media and tease any remaining mesentery/fat off with two sets of forceps.

（4）Collect Peyer's patches by removing them from the intestine with curved scissors and place Peyer's patches in cold harvest media for later isolation steps.

（5）Use the flat side of forceps and gently slide from duodenum towards ileum to expel fecal content and mucus. Repeat once to remove most of the mucus.

（6）Cut the intestine open longitudinally from duodenum to ileum. Laterally cut the opened intestine into 2 cm pieces. Place the intestinal pieces in a 50 mL conical tube with 25 mL cold harvest media for later isolation steps.

2. Isolation of the immune cells from MLE and PP：

（1）Isolate cells from MLN by gently dissociating through a 70 μm cell strainer. Wash cell strainer with 5 mL of cold harvest media.

（2）Pellet MLN-cells by centrifuging at 1,500 r/min for 5 min at 4℃. Resuspend the cell pellet in 1 mL cold harvest media.

（3）Isolate cells from Peyer's patches by incubating Peyer's patches in a 15 mL conical tube containing 5 mL prewarmed collagenase solution at 37℃ and 220 r/min for 30 min on an orbital shaker.

（4）Filter digested tissue and supernatant into a 50 mL conical tube through a 70 μm cell strainer. Gently dissociate the remaining tissue pieces using the plunger of a 3 mL syringe and wash the cell strainer with 5 mL of cold harvest media.

（5）Pellet Peyer's patch cells by centrifuging at 1,500 r/min for 5 min at 4℃ and resuspend the cell pellet in 1 mL cold harvest media.

3. Isolation of intraepithelial immune cells from the intestine：

（1）Wash the pieces of small intestine three times with 25 mL of cold harvest media, let the intestinal pieces settle, and pour off the supernatant.

（2）Add 20 mL of prewarmed DTE solution（DTE is a reducing agent that enriches intraepithelial lymphocytes）to the 50 mL conical tube containing intestine pieces and transfer to a 50 mL siliconized Erlenmeyer flask. Stir at 37℃ and 220 r/min for 20 min and then transfer the tissue and solution back to the 50 mL conical tube.

（3）Vortex the tube at maximum setting for 10 s. Transfer the supernatant into a new 50 mL conical tube through a 70 μm cell strainer, being careful to keep the tissue pieces in the original tube. Do not discard the supernatant; the supernatant contains intraepithelial lymphocytes. Pellet cells by centrifuging at 1,500 r/min for 5 min at 4℃. Resuspend the cell pellet in 10 mL cold harvest media and store on ice.

(4) Repeat step (2) and (3). Transfer the supernatant through a 70 μm cell strainer into the previous tube containing cells from the supernatant of the first DTE treatment (from step (3)).

(5) Pellet cells by centrifuging the supernatant at 1,500 r/min for 5 min at 4℃. Resuspend the cell pellet in 8 mL of 44% DG solution at room temperature (RT).

(6) Transfer the 8 mL 44% DG solution/cell suspension into a 14 mL polypropylene round-bottom tube. Underlay with 5 mL of RT 67% DG solution. Centrifuge at 5 000 r/min for 20 min at RT without using the brake.

(7) Note that viable cells form a band (buffy coat) at the 44% to 67% interface, dead cells and some epithelial cells are in a mucoid film at the top of the gradient, and the red blood cells are in the pellet. Remove the top layer of the gradient to within 2 cm of the interface. Use a Pasteur pipette to harvest the buffy coat at the interface and transfer them to a 50 mL conical tube containing 40 mL cold harvest media.

(8) Pellet cells by centrifuging at 1,500 r/min for 5 min at 4℃. Resuspend the cell pellet in 1 mL cold harvest media.

4. Isolation of lamina propria immune cells from the small intestine:

(1) Remove epithelial cells from intestinal tissue pieces by adding 25 mL of prewarmed EDTA solution (EDTA is a calcium chelator that targets calcium-dependent junctions and promotes the detachment of intestinal epithelial cells) to the flask containing the remaining intestinal pieces. Stir flask at 37℃ and 220 r/min for 30 min and then carefully discard the supernatant while keeping intestinal pieces within the flask.

(2) Repeat step (1).

(3) Add 50 mL of RT harvest media to the flask. Let intestinal pieces settle and carefully discard the supernatant.

(4) Add 30 mL of prewarmed collagenase solution to the flask and stir intestinal pieces at 37℃ and 220 r/min for 45 min.

(5) Transfer digested tissue and supernatant to a 50 mL conical tube by filtering through a 70 μm cell strainer. Gently dissociate remaining tissue pieces by using the plunger of a 3 mL syringe to mash through the filter. Wash the filter with 10 mL of cold harvest media.

(6) Pellet cells by centrifuging at 1,500 r/min for 5 min at 4℃. Resuspend the cell pellet in 8 mL of ambient temperature 44% DG solution.

(7) Transfer the 8 mL 44% DG solution/cell suspension into a 14 mL polypropylene round-bottom tube. Underlay with 5 mL of ambient temperature 67% DG solution. Centrifuge the gradients at 25℃ and 5,000 r/min for 20 min with no brake.

(8) Remove the fat layer on top. Use a Pasteur pipette to harvest the buffy coat at the interface and transfer to a 50 mL conical tube containing 40 mL cold harvest media.

(9) Pellet cells by centrifuging at 1,500 r/min for 5 min at 4℃. Resuspend the cell

pellet in 1 mL cold harvest media.

【Results】

Can obtain a high yield of maximally pure and viable lymphocytes and innate immune cells such as dendritic cells, macrophages, neutrophils, and monocytes. And the isolated immune cells can be subjected to further manipulations like flow cytometric analysis or functional analysis.

【Precautions】

1. It is critical to remove as much mesentery/fat of the intestine as possible for optimal cell yield and viability.

2. Incomplete removal of mucus can decrease cell viability and yield. Nevertheless, be sure to slide the intestine gently to avoid stripping villi or damaging the basement membrane.

3. Red blood cell lysis buffer can be used to remove red blood cells if bleeding occurred.

【Questions】

1. What are the DTE and EDTA used for?
2. What attentions must be paid to in this experiment?

(Shi Junyu   Zheng Fang)

第三篇
Chapter Three

免疫细胞功能检测
Assay for the Functions of Immune Cells

实验二十　　小鼠脾脏 NK 细胞活性检测

【原理】

　　NK 细胞是天然免疫的重要成分。它能产生非特异性的细胞因子和趋化因子等活性物质,无须预先致敏就能裂解靶细胞。大多数肿瘤细胞(如 K562 细胞,YAC－1 细胞)表达的 MHC－I 类分子比正常细胞低,这种 MHC－I 类分子的低表达使由激活性受体结合配体所触发的活化信号超过了由抑制性受体结合 MHC－I 类分子所触发的抑制信号,从而使 NK 细胞活化并攻击靶细胞。我们可以利用 LDH 释放实验检测 NK 细胞对靶细胞的杀伤效应(图 20－1)。

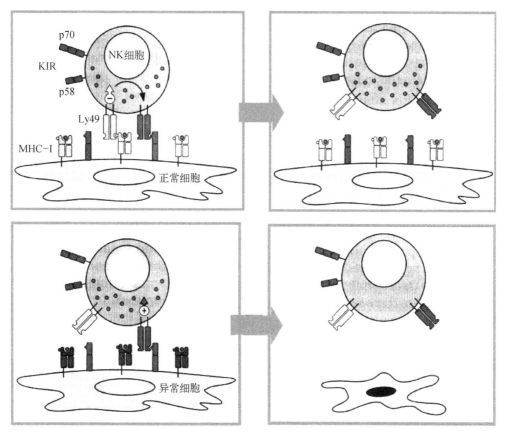

图 20－1　NK 细胞区分并杀伤异常细胞

【应用】

　　检测 NK 细胞活性。如果加入其他细胞因子刺激或者预先用抗原致敏,这一方法亦可用于检测其他细胞活性,如 LAK 或 CTL。

【材料】

1. YAC-1 细胞
2. RPMI-1640 培养液
3. LDH 底物溶液[包括乳酸钠,氧化型辅酶I(NAD$^+$),硝基氯化四氮唑蓝(NBT),吩嗪二甲酯硫酸盐(PMS)]
4. 1% NP-40
5. 细胞培养板、计数板、微量加样器、96 孔板、液氮罐
6. 超净工作台、CO$_2$孵箱、水浴箱
7. 离心机、倒置显微镜、普通光学显微镜、分光光度计

【方法】

1. 靶细胞制备:
(1) 取传代 YAC-1 细胞,于计数板上计数。
(2) 将细胞用 RPMI-1640 培养液调至 1×10^{6}细胞/mL 浓度供实验用。

2. 效应细胞制备:
(1) 断椎处死小鼠,浸于 70% 乙醇中 10 min。暴露并在无菌环境下取出脾脏放入平皿中。
(2) 将脾用镊子在钢丝网上磨碎,于 2 mL 培养液中静置 5 min,取无沉渣液,或直接用纱布块过滤,1 500 r/min 离心 10 min。
(3) 弃上清后,用 3 mL 无菌蒸馏水裂解红细胞 40 s,用 1 mL 3.6% 的盐水恢复等渗。重悬细胞。
(4) 2 000 r/min 离心 10 min,弃上清,用培养液调至所需浓度。

3. 效靶细胞反应:取效应细胞及靶细胞各 100 μL 加入 96 孔板中,效靶比为 100∶1;自然释放组为靶细胞和 RPMI-1640 培养液各 100 μL;最大释放组为靶细胞和 1% NP-40 各 100 μL。每组设两个平行复孔(表 20-1)。孵育 2~4 h。转出上清 100 μL/孔至新孔,每孔加入 LDH 底物溶液(图 20-2)100 μL,室温避光孵育 10~15 min,加入 1 mol/L 的柠檬酸溶液 50 μL 终止反应。在 570 nm 处读取各组 OD 值。

表 20-1   效靶细胞混合

	实验组(t)		自然释放组(n)		最大释放组(m)	
	1	2	3	4	5	6
靶细胞(YAC-1)(100 μL)	+	+	+	+	+	+
效应(NK)细胞 (100 μL)	+	+	-	-	-	-
RPMI-1640 (100 μL)	-	-	+	+	-	-
1% NP-40 (100 μL)	-	-	-	-	+	+

【结果】

NK 细胞杀伤活性(%)=[1-(杀伤孔 OD-效应孔 OD)/靶细胞孔 OD]×100%

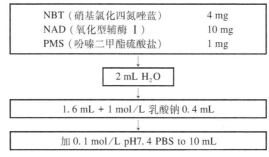

图 20-2　LDH 底物溶液的配制

【注意事项】

1. 靶细胞状态要良好,一般传代时间超过 2 个月的 YAC-1 细胞不应作靶细胞,需重新从液氮罐中取出复苏。

2. 效靶细胞混合要充分。

3. 实验中一定要设置自然释放组。

【思考题】

1. NK 细胞杀伤靶细胞与 CTL 杀伤靶细胞作用机制有何不同?

2. NK 细胞对靶细胞的杀伤效应还可以用其他什么方法进行检测?

（郑　芳）

Exp. 20   Mouse Spleen NK Cells Activity Assay

【**Principle**】

Natural killer (NK) cells are crucial components of the innate immune system. NK cells can produce non-specific cytokines and chemokines, and have ability to lyse target cells without prior sensitization. Most tumor cells such as K562 cells or YAC‐1 express less MHC class‐I molecules on their surfaces than the normal cells. And this lost of MHC class-I allows activating signals, which are triggered by activating receptors binding to ligands, to overcome inhibition signals, which are triggered by inhibitory receptors binding to MHC class-I molecules. Then we can use LDH release assay to determine the cytotoxicity of NK cells(Fig.20‐1).

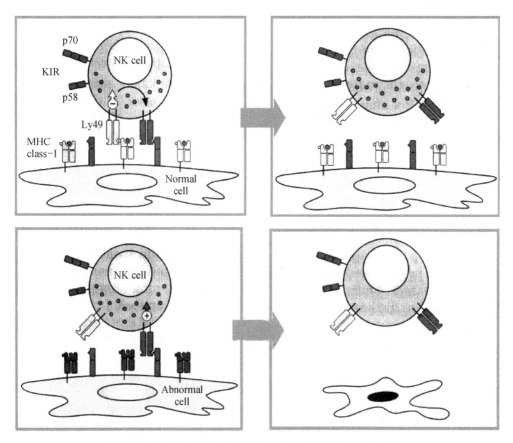

Fig.20‐1   How NK cells distinguish and kill abnormal cells

【**Application**】

Determination of NK cell activity. This test can also be used to detect other cellular activities, such as LAK or CTL, if sensitization with cytokine antigen stimulation.

【Materials】

1. YAC – 1 cells

2. RPMI – 1640 culture medium

3. LDH substrate solution: lactic acid, nicotinamide-adenine dinucleotide (NAD$^+$), nitroblue tetrazolium (NBT), PMS

4. 1% NP – 40

5. Cell culture flasks, liquid nitrogen can, cytometer, pipettes, 96-well plates, hemocytometer

6. Super clean bench, CO$_2$ incubator, water bath

7. Centrifuge, invert microscopes and light microscopes, spectrophotometer

【Procedures】

1. Preparation of target cells

(1) YAC – 1 cells are subcultured for 24 h and counted on the cytometer.

(2) Adjust cell concentration to about 1×10^6 cells/mL with supplemented RPMI –1640.

2. Preparation of effector cells

(1) A mouse is sacrificed. Put the mouse into 70% alcohol for 10 minutes. Expose and take out the spleen sterilely and put it in a plate.

(2) Pound the spleen into pieces with forceps. Then put the spleen pieces into a tube with 2 ml culture medium for 5 min. Collect the suspension without dregs or filter the mixture with gauze. The collected solution is centrifuged at 1,500 r/min for 10 min.

(3) The supernatant is discarded. Lyse RBCs by adding 3 mL sterile distilled water into the tube and stand for 40 s. Then add 1 mL 3.6% saline solution to resume isotonic state and stop lysis. Then resuspend cells.

(4) Centrifuge cell suspension at 2,000 r/min for 10 min and discard supernatant. Cells are resuspended and adjusted to needed concentration with culture medium.

3. Reaction of effector and target: A 96-well plate is divided into such groups: test group — 100 μL effect cells and 100 μL target cells are added into each well, and ratio of them is 100 : 1; nature release group—100 μL target cells and 100 μL RPMI – 1640 are added into each well; maximum release group — 100 μL target cells and 100 μL 1% NP40 are added into each well(Tab.20 – 1). All groups are incubated at incubator for 2 – 4 h. Then transfer 100 μL supernatant to the empty well in turn, add 100 μL fresh LDH substrate solution (Fig.20 – 2) to the well, incubate 10 – 15 minutes at room temperature in darkness, and terminate the reaction with 1M citric acid (50 μL)

Tab.20 - 1   Mixing of target cell and effect cell

	test(t)		natural release(n)		maximum release(m)	
	1	2	3	4	5	6
Target cell (YAC - 1)(100 μL)	+	+	+	+	+	+
Effect (NK) cell (100 μL)	+	+	-	-	-	-
RPMI - 1640 (100 μL)	-	-	+	+	-	-
1% NP - 40 (100 μL)	-	-	-	-	+	+

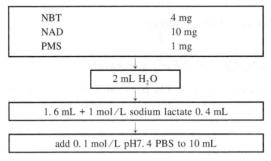

Fig.20 - 2   Preparation of LDH substrate solution

【Results】

NK cell activity = [1 - (OD$_C$ - OD$_E$)/OD$_T$] × 100%

OD$_C$: OD value from cytotoxic cells group.

OD$_E$: OD value from effection cells group.

OD$_T$: OD value from target cells group.

【Precautions】

1. Target cells must be kept in good state. YAC - 1 subcultured for more than 2 months should be discarded. Use new cells resuscitated from liquid nitrogen.

2. Effect cells and target cells must be mixed sufficiently to get complete reaction.

3. Natural release group is necessary.

【Questions】

1. What is the difference between the action mechanism of NK cells and CTL cells?

2. Is there any other method used to detect the killing effect of NK cells on target cells?

(Zheng Fang)

实验二十一　豚鼠 T 细胞 E 玫瑰花环试验

【原理】

豚鼠 T 淋巴细胞表面具有兔红细胞受体,在体外一定条件下,豚鼠 T 淋巴细胞能直接与兔红细胞(RRBC)结合,形成玫瑰花样细胞团,称为 E 玫瑰花环。为保证有足够的 T 淋巴细胞,取豚鼠的胸腺做 E 玫瑰花环试验(图 21-1)。

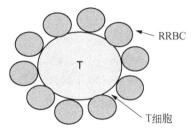

图 21-1　E 玫瑰花环形成示意图

【应用】

检测外周血或胸腺中 T 淋巴细胞数目。

【材料】

1. 无 Ca^{2+}、Mg^{2+} HBSS
2. Alsever's 保存液
3. 1% 兔红细胞悬液
4. 0.8% 戊二醛溶液
5. 胎牛血清(FCS)
6. 甲紫染液
7. 剪刀、镊子、铜网、平皿、研磨棒、吸管、试管、离心机、显微镜等

【方法】

1. 淋巴细胞悬液的制备:

(1)铜网置于平皿中。

(2)取胸腺:断颈法处死豚鼠,仰卧位固定于蜡盘,剪开豚鼠颈部皮肤,暴露其下的透明胸膜,可见透明胸膜下气管上两侧各有一蚕豆大小的胸腺。用镊子夹住胸腺,全部取下,置于铜网上。剪开胸腺,将其剖面在载玻片上涂几下,加一滴甲紫染液,显微镜下观察。

(3)研磨法制备胸腺单细胞悬液:在胸腺上滴加 1 mL HBSS,用玻璃注射器柱塞轻轻研磨,使胸腺细胞穿过铜网漏入平皿中。用少量 HBSS 将黏附在柱塞和铜网上的细胞冲下,吸取细胞悬液于塑料试管中。

(4)洗涤细胞:补加约 8 mL HBSS,吹打混匀洗涤细胞,配平后,1 500 r/min,离心 5 min。

(5)调整细胞浓度:弃上清,用 Hank's 液定容到 3 mL,吹打混匀,细胞浓度约为 3×10^6 细胞/mL。

2. 兔红细胞悬液的制备:

取一定量 Alsever's 保存液保存的兔红细胞于试管中,用无 Ca^{2+}、Mg^{2+} HBSS 离心、洗涤 3 次,前 2 次均以 2 000 r/min 离心 5 min;第 3 次以 2 000 r/min 离心 10 min。取上述细胞沉淀用 HBSS 配成 1% 细胞悬液(细胞浓度约为 $2×10^8$ 细胞/mL)。

3. E 玫瑰花环的形成:

(1) 取一支塑料试管,加入 0.5 mL 淋巴细胞悬液,0.5 mL 1% 兔红细胞悬液、1 滴胎牛血清(保护细胞),混匀。

(2) 配平后,以 500 r/min 离心 5 min。

(3) 吸弃 1/2 上清,加 0.8% 戊二醛 1 滴(固定作用,防成花细胞分离),轻轻旋转试管,小心混匀。取 1 滴细胞悬液,滴于载玻片,加 1 滴甲紫染液,盖上盖玻片,低倍镜下找到视野,高倍镜下观察。

【结果】

一般结合 3 个以上兔红细胞者为 1 个 E 玫瑰花环阳性细胞,计数 200 个淋巴细胞中形成 E 玫瑰花环的淋巴细胞百分数。

【注意事项】

1. 试验中所用的兔红细胞必须新鲜。
2. 计数前重悬细胞时,动作要轻,不可用力震摇或强力吹打,以免花环消失。
3. 兔红细胞与淋巴细胞比例以 100:1 为宜。

【思考题】

为何要用新鲜的血标本测 E 玫瑰花环?

(曾瑞红)

Exp. 21　Erythrocyte Rosette Forming Cell Test (ERFC) for Guinea Pig T Cells

【Principle】

The surface of guinea pig T lymphocyte contains the receptor of rabbit erythrocyte. Under certain conditions in vitro, guinea pig T lymphocytes can directly bind to rabbit red blood cells (RRBC) to form E rosette by its E receptor (Fig.21 - 1).

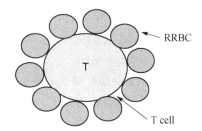

Fig.21 - 1　Schematic illustration of E-rosette

【Application】

This test is used to detect the number of T lymphocytes from peripheral blood or thymus.

【Materials】

1. Ca^{2+} and Mg^{2+} free Hank's Balanced Salt Solution (HBSS)
2. Alsever's preservative solution
3. 1% rabbit erythrocyte
4. 0.8% glutaraldehyde water solution
5. Fetal calf serum (FCS)
6. methylrosanilnium chloride solution
7. Scissors, forceps, copper mesh, plates, grinding rods, pipette, test tube, centrifuge, microscope, etc.

【Procedures】

1. Preparation for lymphocyte suspension:

(1) Place the copper mesh on the plate.

(2) Take the thymus: the guinea pig is killed by breaking the neck and fixed on the wax dish in supine position. Cut the neck skin, exposing the transparent membrane. There is a bean-sized thymus on each side of the trachea. Hold the thymus with forceps, cut them all, and place them on the copper mesh. Cut the thymus, smear its profile on the glass slide, add a drop of methylrosanilnium chloride solution, observe under the microscope.

(3) Thymocyte suspension is prepared by grinding: add 1 mL HBSS to the thymus and gently ground with a glass grinding rods to allow thymocytes to pass through the copper mesh into the plate. The cells attaching to the rods and the copper mesh are washed with a small amount of HBSS, and the cell suspension is pipetted into a plastic test tube.

(4) Wash the cells: add 8 mL HBSS, mix well, centrifuge at 1,500 r/min for 5 min.

(5) Adjust the thymocyte concentration: decant the supernatant, add HBSS to make 3 mL cell suspension, mix well, and the cell concentration is about 3×10^6 cells/mL.

2. Preparation for rabbit erythrocyte suspension:

Wash rabbit erythrocyte for three times in Ca^{2+} and Mg^{2+} free Hank's Balanced Salt Solution. For the first and second time, centrifuge at 2,000 r/min for 5 min. In the third time, centrifuge at 2,000 r/min for 10 min. Aspirate 0.1 mL cell pellet and adjust cell suspension to 2×10^8 cells/mL using Hank's Balanced Salt Solution to make 1% rabbit erythrocyte suspension.

3. Formation of E-rosette:

(1) Aspirate 0.5 mL of lymphocyte suspension, 0.5 mL of 1% of rabbit erythrocyte suspension and a drop of fetal calf serum (protect the cells) into a test tube. Mix gently.

(2) Centrifuge at 500 r/min for 5 min.

(3) Aspirate 1/2 supernatant, add a drop of 0.8% glutaraldehyde water solution (fixation, prevent E-rosette from separating), gently rotate the tube and mix carefully. Add a drop of cell suspension and a drop of methylrosanilnium chloride solution to a microslide, put a cover glass. Observe the rosette forming cells under the microscope.

【Results】

The percentage of E-rosette formation is calculated by counting the rosette forming cells of 200 viable lymphocytes. The lymphocyte is scored as a rosette forming cell if three or more erythrocytes are adherent to one lymphocyte.

【Precautions】

1. The rabbit erythrocyte suspension must be fresh.

2. Must not shake after E-rosette formation to prevent E-rosette falling away.

3. It is the best for rabbit erythrocyte and lymphocyte in the proportion of 100 : 1.

【Question】

Why use the fresh blood sample to measure the E-rosette?

(Zeng Ruihong)

实验二十二 SAP 酶标法测定 T 细胞亚群

【原理】

利用免疫酶标记技术检测淋巴细胞的表面标志,对 T 细胞及其亚群进行鉴定。首先用鼠抗人 T 细胞 CD 分子的 IgG 类单克隆抗体(Ab1)与 T 细胞表面相应的 CD 分子结合,再用生物素(biotin)标记的羊抗小鼠 IgG(Ab2)孵育,然后利用生物素-链霉亲和素高效结合的特点,加入碱性磷酸酶标记的链霉卵白素(streptavidin/alkaline phosphatase,SAP),最后通过酶促底物反应显色以检测 CD 分子,从而鉴定 T 细胞及 T 细胞亚群(图 22-1)。

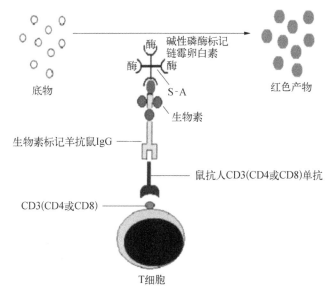

图 22-1 SAP 酶标法测定 T 细胞亚群示意图

【应用】

因抗体可连接多个生物素,1 个链霉亲和素具有 4 个亚基,其中一个亚基结合生物素,其余 3 个可结合多个酶,组成生物放大系统,提高了检测的敏感性。

【材料】

1. 常规分离外周血单个核细胞材料
2. HBSS 或 RPMI-1640 培养液、PBS
3. 防脱片剂
4. 固定剂
5. 一抗(IgG):小鼠抗人 CD3 单抗,小鼠抗人 CD4 单抗,小鼠抗人 CD8 单抗;二抗:生物素标记羊抗小鼠 IgG(IgG/Bio)

6. 碱性磷酸酶标记链霉卵白素（SAP）

7. 显色剂（底物）

8. 细胞核复染剂

9. 载玻片、细胞计数板、试管、巴斯德吸管、离心机、温箱等

【方法】

1. 取防脱剂 5~10 μL 滴加在载玻片上均匀推片，亦可用棉签黏取防脱片剂均匀涂于干净玻片上，待干后制备细胞涂片，以防脱片。

2. 常规分离外周血单个核细胞（PBMC）。沉积的 PBMC 利用试管中剩余的少许回流液体（约 1 滴）混匀细胞，制成单个核细胞悬液。取 30 μL 细胞悬液滴于载玻片上，静止 2 min 使细胞下沉黏附于玻片上，吸去液体，快速吹干（或用 PBS 将单个核细胞调至 $2×10^5$ 个/mL，离心涂片机 1 000 r/min 离心 1~2 min 制片，快速吹干，或 37℃温箱 1 h 烤干）。

3. 充分干燥的细胞涂片先用记号笔在标本外画圈（在载玻片背面画），然后滴加固定剂 50 μL，室温静止 2~3 min，用 PBS 淋洗，擦干玻片背面及细胞外的 PBS。

4. 分别滴加小鼠抗人 CD3（或 CD4，或 CD8）单抗 IgG 适量（10~30 μL），湿盒中 37℃孵育 30 min（或 4℃过夜），PBS 淋洗 3 次。

5. 滴加生物素标记的羊抗小鼠 IgG 适量（10~30 μL），湿盒中 37℃孵育 30~45 min，PBS 淋洗 3 次。

6. 滴加碱性磷酸酶标记链霉卵白素（SAP）适量（10~30 μL），湿盒中 37℃孵育 30~45 min，PBS 淋洗 3 次。

7. 滴加显色剂 30~50 μL，室温显色 20~40 min。在显微镜下观察，待细胞膜上出现红色标记物时，用 PBS 淋洗。

8. 滴加细胞核复染液 30~50 μL，30 s 后用自来水淋洗。

【结果】

高倍镜下选取染色好的视野计数 100~200 个单个核细胞，细胞表面有红色标记物为阳性细胞。算出阳性率。

外周人血中，阳性细胞百分率的正常参考值：CD3，60%~80%；CD4，35%~55%；CD8，20%~30%；CD4/CD8 值为 1.5~2.0。

【注意事项】

1. 制备涂片时细胞数不能过多。

2. 所用玻片须涂过防脱片剂，细胞染色前须经过固定。

【思考题】

如何用 SAP 法检测 B 细胞亚群？

（王　瑾　屈子璐）

Exp. 22   Detection of T Lymphocyte Subgroups in Peripheral Blood by the SAP

【Principle】

     The surface markers of lymphocytes are detected by immunoenzymatic technique to identify T cells and their subgroups. Firstly, the IgG monoclonal antibody (Ab1) of mouse anti-human T cell CD molecule is combined with CD molecule on T cell surface, then goat anti-mouse IgG labeled with biotin (Ab2) is added. Due to the highly affinity of biotin with streptavidin, added streptavidin labeled with alkali phosphatase (SAP) can bind with biotin. Finally, the CD molecule is detected by enzymatic substrate reaction, so as to identify T and T cell subgroups(Fig.22 − 1).

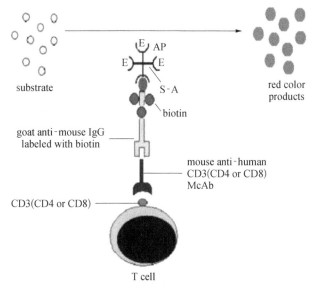

Fig.22 − 1   Schematic diagram of SAP reaction

【Application】

     Antibodies can be linked to a number of biotin. One streptavidin has four subunits. One subunit combines with biotin, and the other three subunits can combine with multiple enzymes. The above interaction forms a biological amplification system to improve the sensitivity of detection.

【Materials】

     1. The materials of separated peripheral blood mononuclear cell

2. HBSS or RPMI – 1640 medium, PBS

3. Adhesion solution

4. Fixed agent

5. Primary antibodies (IgG): mouse anti-human CD3 monoclonal antibody, mouse anti-human CD4 monoclonal antibody, mouse anti-human CD8 monoclonal antibody. Secondary antibody: goat anti-mouse IgG labeled with biotin

6. Streptavidin labeled with alkali phosphatase (SAP)

7. Substrate solution

8. Nuclear stain

9. Glass slide, cell counting chamber, test tube, Pasteur pipette, centrifuges, humidified incubator, etc.

【Procedures】

1. Glass slide should be pre-treated by smearing 5 – 10 μL adhesion solution and dried before adding the cell suspension.

2. PBMCs are separated from whole blood (reference exp. 18). After discarding the suspension, leave one drop of medium and resuspend the cells in the bottom. Add 30 μL PBMC suspension onto the treated slide, wait 2 minutes and let the cells adhere to the slide, draw liquid away and dry it by blowing fleetly or roasting at 37℃ (or adjust the cell concentration at 2×10^5 cells/mL in PBS, 1,000 r/min for 1 – 2 min by cytocentrifugation and also dry it by blowing fleetly or roasting at 37℃).

3. Draw the sample area on the back of the fully dried cell smear using a marker pen, add 50 μL fixation solution and wait for 2 – 3 min at room temperature. Wash the slide by PBS and dry the back of the slide and outside the marked area.

4. Add mouse anti-human CD3 (CD4 or CD8) monoclonal antibodies (10 – 30 μL) into the cell area, incubate at 37℃ for 30 min (or 4℃ overnight), and wash it by PBS for 3 times.

5. Add goat anti-mouse IgG labeled with biotin (10 – 30 μL), incubate for at 37℃ 30 – 45 min in the wet box, and wash it for 3 times.

6. Add 10 – 30 μL streptavidin labeled with alkali phosphatase (SAP) and incubate at 37℃ for 30 min, and wash the slide for 3 times.

7. Add 30 – 50 μL substrate complex onto the slide and react at room temperature for 20 – 40 min, and observe it by microscope. The red colour appears on the cell membrane, wash it by PBS immediately.

8. Add 30 – 50 μL nuclear stain for 30s, and wash it by water.

【Results】

The percentage of positive cells are calculated by counting 100 – 200 cells in field of vision, and the positive cell is stained red on the membrane.

The normal referenced values of positive cells in PBMC: CD3, 60%−80%; CD4, 35%−55%; CD8, 20%−30%; the ratio of CD4/CD8 is 1. 5 − 2. 0.

【Precautions】

1. Don't add too many cells to make smear.

2. The slides should be coated with adherent solution and the cells need be fixed before staining.

【Question】

How to detect B cell subgroups by SAP?

(Wang Jin   Qu Zilu)

实验二十三 单向混合淋巴细胞反应

【原理】

同种间或异种间两个不同个体的淋巴细胞在体外混合培养,能相互刺激而发生增殖反应,称为双向混合淋巴细胞反应(MLR)或混合淋巴细胞培养(MLC)。将两个不同个体之一的淋巴细胞经丝裂霉素C(阻止DNA合成)或X线照射处理,抑制其增殖能力而保持抗原性,以这些细胞作为刺激细胞,将另一个不经过处理的细胞作为反应细胞,两者进行混合培养。在2~3天内,刺激细胞引起反应细胞转化(增加DNA合成)成淋巴母细胞,此反应为单向MLR。培养5天后,加入 ^3H-胸腺嘧啶核苷(^3H-TdR,一种DNA的放射性前体),再经16~20 h培养后测定同位素掺入。 ^3H-TdR掺入量反映了细胞上MHC II 的不匹配程度(图23-1)。

【应用】

MLR主要用于组织移植前受者与供者组织抗原的配型检测,也可以作为研究免疫调节的细胞实验模型。

【材料】

1. 小鼠脾细胞
2. 丝裂霉素C
3. RPMI-1640完全培养液(含20% NCS)
4. ^3H-胸腺嘧啶核苷
5. Hank's
6. 闪烁液
7. 玻璃纤维滤纸
8. 液闪管
9. 干燥箱
10. 细胞收集器
11. 液闪计数仪
12. 96孔培养板、吸管、吸头、孵育箱等

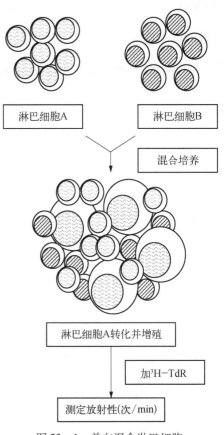

图23-1 单向混合淋巴细胞
反应示意图

【方法】

1. 制备取自两个不同品系小鼠(C57 和 BALB/c)的脾细胞。

2. BALB/c 脾细胞在 37℃ 中用丝裂霉素 C(最终浓度为 25~50 mg/mL)处理 30 min,1 000 r/min 离心 10 min,用 Hank's 液洗涤 2~3 次,作为刺激细胞(淋巴细胞 B);未经丝裂霉素 C 处理的 C57 脾细胞作为反应细胞(淋巴细胞 A)。用完全 RPMI-1640 培养液调整细胞浓度至 $2×10^6$ 个/mL。

3. 将反应细胞(A)和刺激细胞(B)各 0.1 mL 加入 96 孔细胞培养板的微孔内(每孔 $2×10^5$ 细胞),同时设置未刺激培养对照,均做三个复孔,置 37℃、5% CO_2 培养箱内培养 5 天。

4. 于培养终止前 16 h 每孔加入 ^3H-TdR 1 μCi。

5. 培养结束后,借助于细胞收集器将标记有同位素的样品收集于玻璃纤维滤纸上,用生理盐水洗去游离同位素。

6. 将玻璃纤维滤纸放人干燥箱中烘干,再置于含有闪烁液的液闪管中,用 β 液体闪烁计数仪测定放射性(cpm 值)。

【结果】

有两种基本的结果表示方法:

1. 计算刺激的和未刺激的(对照)培养中每种处理三个复孔的 cpm 平均值。

2. 按照以下公式算出刺激指数(SI):

$$SI = 被刺激细胞平均 cpm / 相应对照细胞平均 cpm。$$

【注意事项】

1. 丝裂霉素 C 处理后,用 Hank's 液洗涤细胞 3 次,清除丝裂霉素 C。

2. MLC 终止时,用细胞收集器以生理盐水彻底洗涤细胞,去除游离的 ^3H-TdR。

3. 实验操作需在无菌条件下进行。

4. 避免 ^3H 污染环境,采取防辐射措施。

【思考题】

测出的 cpm 值比对照明显升高说明什么?

(田野平)

Exp. 23　　One-way Mixed Lymphocyte Reaction

【Principle】

A proliferation reaction is obtained when lymphocytes taken from two homogeneous or from two heterogeneous individuals are mixed *in vitro* culture. This reaction is known as the two-way mixed lymphocyte reaction (MLR) or mixed lymphocyte culture (MLC). A cell sample from each individual is treated with either mitomycin C (to block DNA synthesis) or X-irradiation in order to arrest proliferative ability and maintain antigenicity. These treated cells are used as stimulators in culture with untreated cells, responders. Stimulators cause responders to transform (with increase of DNA synthesis) into lymphoblasts within 2 to 3 days. This reaction is the one-way MLR. After 4 to 5 days culture, ^{3}H-thymidine (a radioactive precursor of DNA) is added. After an additional 16 to 20 h incubation, the incorporation of the isotope into DNA is determined. The uptake of ^{3}H-thymidine reflects the mismatching extent of MHC – Ⅱ antigens on cells (Fig.23 – 1).

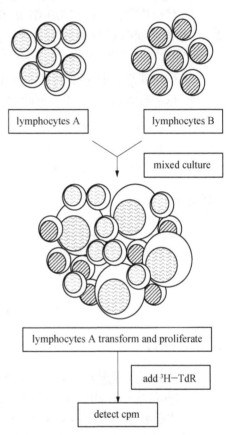

Fig.23 – 1　One-way mixed lymphocyte

【Application】

MLR is mainly applied for matching of tissue antigens from recipient and donor before tissue transplantation. MLR may also be applied for study immune regulation as a cellular experiment model.

【Materials 】

1. Mouse splenocytes
2. Mitomycin C
3. Complete RPMI – 1640 medium containing 20% NCS
4. ^{3}H-thymidine
5. Hank's solution

6. Scintillation liquid

7. Glass fiber filter

8. Scintillation vials

9. Drying oven

10. Cell harvester

11. Liquid scintillation counter

12. 96 - well culture plate, pipettes, tips, incubator, etc.

【Procedures】

1. Prepare splenocyte suspensions from two outbred mice (C57BL/6 J and BALB/c).

2. Treat the BALB/c splenocytes with mitomycin C (25 - 50 μg/mL) at 37℃ for 30 min, centrifuge at 1,000 r/min for 10 min and wash the cells three times with Hank's solution. These cells are used as MLR stimulator cells (lymphocyte B). Splenocytes of C57BL/6 J, untreated by mitomycin C are used as MLR responder cells (lymphocyte A). Adjust to 2×10^6 cells/mL with complete RPMI - 1640 medium.

3. Prepare MLR cultures using lymphocyte A and lymphocyte B. Mix 0. 1 mL each type of cells into 96-well culture plate (2×10^5 cells per well) and set up the unstimulated culture control spontaneously. Add triplicates of each treatment and culture at 37℃ for 5 days.

4. Add 1 μ Ci ^{3}H-thymidine to each culture on the 5th day of the MLR and culture continually for 16 h.

5. Collect the cells using the harvester, transfer them from the wells to the glass fiber filters and wash the cells three times with saline.

6. Dry the glass fiber filters thoroughly in a drying oven and deposit them in the scintillation vials. Add 1 mL scintillation liquid into each vial for counting cpm by a liquid scintillation counter.

【Results】

There are basically two methods of result presentation:

1. Calculate the mean cpm count for triplicates of each treatment in simulated and unstimulated (control) cultures.

2. Calculate a stimulating index according to the formula, stimulating index (SI) = mean cpm of the stimulated cells/mean cpm of the corresponding control cells.

【Precautions】

1. Wash the cells three times after mitomycin C treatment with Hank's solution to clean out mitomycin C.

2. Wash the cells thoroughly at the end of MLC with saline using the harvester to clean out free ^{3}H-thymidine.

3. The experimental operation should be proceeded in an aseptic condition.

4. Avoid the environment to be contaminated by^{3}H. Take the protective measure against radiation.

【Question】

Please explain why the measured cpm value is higher than the control?

(Tian Yeping)

实验二十四　　细胞毒性 T 细胞活性测定

【原理】

细胞毒性 T 淋巴细胞(CTL)具有抗原特异性的细胞毒活性,可杀伤带有特异性抗原的靶细胞,在宿主针对肿瘤、移植物和病毒的免疫反应中发挥重要作用。

MHC 限制性的 CTL 的细胞毒活性通常是用与实验鼠来源于同一品系、经多肽刺激、病毒感染或修饰后的小鼠肿瘤细胞系(如 P815[H－2^d])作为靶细胞,效应细胞和刺激细胞则来自实验鼠脾单细胞悬液(为 B 细胞、巨噬细胞、树突状细胞及 CTL 等细胞的混合物)。

靶细胞裂解由 ^{51}Cr 释放测定。当被标记的抗原靶细胞被 CTL 杀伤后,胞内的 ^{51}Cr 即释入上清中,^{51}Cr 的释放量可定量检测,经与对照孔比较,得到 ^{51}Cr 的释放率,据此判断 CTL 的功能活性。

【应用】

作为评价机体抗原特异性 CTL 活性的一个指标。

【材料】

1. RPMI－1640 完全培养液
2. RPMI－2:含 2% FCS 的 RPMI－1640 培养液
3. 1% Triton X－100
4. IL－2、Na^{51}CrO$_4$
5. 靶细胞

【方法】

1. 用脾单细胞作为鼠 CTL 效应细胞和刺激细胞:

(1) 制备病毒感染或免疫后小鼠的脾单细胞,用完全培养液,调整细胞浓度为 2×10^6 个/mL。

(2) 根据试验目的,分别用活病毒(病毒用量因病毒而异,如痘苗病毒重组体的用量为 1~5 PFU/细胞),或特异性多肽(应为与免疫鼠时相同的多肽,1 μg/mL),在 50 mL 烧瓶(直立)中与脾单细胞一起于 37℃、CO$_2$ 培养箱中共同孵育,反应体积 10~20 mL。

(3) 培养后 3~4 d,向反应体系中加入 IL－2 至 5 U/mL,继续培养 4~5 d。如换液及补充 IL－2 后,可延长培养时间。

(4) 培养结束后,1 500 r/min 离心 5 min,进行活细胞计数。

(5) 用完全培养液,调整细胞浓度为 2×10^6~4×10^6 个/mL。

2. 制备 ^{51}Cr 标记的靶细胞:

(1) 取 5×10^6 靶细胞,离心,重悬于 0.2~0.3 mL 无血清的培养液中。

(2) 加入 100 μCi^{51}Cr/5×10^{6}细胞,于 37℃孵育 60 min。

(3) 加入 10 mL、RPMI-2,离心(1 500 r/min,5 min),弃上清至放射性物质废物容器内。重复两次。

(4) 用完全培养液重悬细胞,计数活细胞数。

(5) 调整细胞浓度为 2×10^{5}个/mL。

3. CTL 活性分析:

(1) 加入抗原(用量因抗原而异)到靶细胞中,共同孵育 2 h,洗两次,调整细胞浓度为 2×10^{5}细胞/mL。

(2) 用完全培养液,按 2×稀释法,制备效应细胞,用多通道加样器加入 96 孔培养板中,每个稀释度做 3 个复孔。

(3) 加入 100 μL 靶细胞到相应的效应细胞孔及另外的 12 个不含有效应细胞的孔中,其中的 6 个孔加入 100 μL 完全培养液,用以测定靶细胞^{51}Cr 自发释放,另外的 6 个孔加入 100 μL 1%(V/V)的 Triton X-100,用以测定靶细胞的^{51}Cr 最大释放量。

(4) 将 96 孔板置于离心吊篮上,离心(1 000 r/min,1 min),聚集效、靶细胞于孔底,利于互相作用。

(5) 37℃,孵育 4~6 h。

(6) 1 500 r/min 离心 5 min。

(7) 用多通道加样器收集各孔上清 100 μL 于一新的培养板中,以测定上清的 cpm 值。

【结果】

特异性释放(%)=[(实验孔 cpm-自发释放孔 cpm/最大释放孔 cpm-自发释放孔 cpm)]×100

【注意事项】

如果自发释放孔>20%,该次实验结果无效。

【思考题】

本实验所用的效应细胞为脾脏单细胞悬液,如用脾脏单细胞悬液制备的淋巴细胞作为效应细胞,该实验应如何进行?

(何金生)

Exp. 24   Measurement of CTL Activity

【Principle】

Cytotoxic T lymphocytes (CTL) have antigen-specific cytotoxicity activity. They can kill target cells on the basis of cell-surface antigen recognition, and are important in the host responses to tumors, transplants, and viruses.

The MHC-restricted cytotoxic activity of CTL is usually measured by the use of peptide-pulsed, virus-infected or modified murine tumor cell lines as target cells, which are MHC-compatible with the responding T-cell (e. g. , P815[$H - 2^d$]). The CTL effector cells and the stimulator cells can be prepared with responder mouse spleen single-cell suspensions (mixtures of B-cells, macrophages, dendritic cells and CTL, etc.).

The lysis of target cells is determined by the chromium-release assay. The labelled antigenic targets are recognized and lysed, and release radioactivity into the supernatant. The amount of ^{51}Cr released into the supernatant is quantitated. By comparison with ^{51}Cr release of controls, the percentage cytotoxicity is calculated for each concentration of effector cells.

【Application】

Be used as an appraisal index of the antigen-specific CTL activity.

【Materials】

1. RPMI – 1640 complete medium
2. RPMI – 2: RPMI – 1640 medium supplemented with 2% (V/V) FCS
3. 1% Triton X – 100
4. IL – 2, Na^{51}CrO$_4$
5. Target cells

【Procedures】

1. Preparation of murine CTL effector and stimulator cells from spleen cells:

(1) Prepare spleen single-cell suspension from virus-infected or immunized mice, and suspend at 2×10^6 cells/mL in complete medium.

(2) Culture cells with live virus (concentration to be established for each virus, e. g. vaccinia virus recombinant 1 – 5 PFU/cell), or specific peptide (1 μg/mL; previously shown to be recognized by mice of the corresponding haplotype) in 10 – 20 mL vol in 50 mL flasks (upright) at 37℃ in a CO$_2$ incubator.

(3) Add 5 U/mL of IL－2 after 3－4 d and culture for a further 4－5 d or longer if fresh medium and IL－2 are added.

(4) At the end of the culture period, centrifuge cells (1,500 r/min, 5 min), and count the number of viable cells.

(5) Resuspend at $(2-4)\times10^{6}$ cells/mL in complete medium.

2. Preparation of ^{51}Cr-labeled target cells:

(1) Centrifuge 5×10^{6} target cells and resuspend in 0.2－0.3 mL of serum-free medium.

(2) Add 100 μCi^{51}Cr/5×10^{6} cells and incubate for 60 min at 37℃.

(3) Add 10 mL of RPMI－2, centrifuge(1,500 r/min,5 min), and discard supernatant into radioactive waster container. Repeat twice.

(4) Resuspend in complete medium and count the number of viable cells.

(5) Resuspend at 2×10^{5} cells /mL.

3. CTL activity assay:

(1) Add antigen (the optimum concentrations to be determined for individual antigens) to the target cells and incubate them together for 2 h. Then wash twice, and resuspend to 2×10^{5} cells/mL.

(2) Prepare twofold dilutions of the effector cells in complete medium in triplicate wells of 96-wells plates using a multichannel pipet.

(3) Add 100 μL of target cells to each of the wells with effector cells and 12 additional wells without effector cells. Add 100 μL complete medium to 6 of these wells to measure spontaneous^{51}Cr release from target cells, and 100 μL of 1%(V/V)Triton X－100 to the other 6 wells to measure maxium^{51}Cr release from target cells.

(4) Use plate carriers, centrifuge the plate(s) (1,000 r/min,1 min) to pellet the cells gently and allow interaction of CTL effector and target cells.

(5) Incubate at 37℃ for 4－6 h.

(6) Centrifuge the plate(s) for 5 min at 1 500 r/min.

(7) Harvest 100 μL of supernatant from each well by using a multichannel pipet, and transfer them to a fresh plate for counting.

【Results】

Calculate the percentage of cytotoxicity using the average values of the replicates from the experimental (E), spontaneous release (S) and maximum release (M) as follows:

$$[(E-S)/(M-S)] \times 100$$

【Precautions】

If spontaneous release is >20%, the results may not be reliable.

【Question】

In this experiment, the murine spleen single-cell suspension is used as the effector cells when the lymphocytes from splenocytes are used as effector cells, how do you formulate your experimental design?

(He Jinsheng)

第四篇
Chapter Four

抗体制备
Preparation of Antibody

实验二十五　多克隆抗体的制备

【原理】

将可溶性抗原和颗粒性抗原注入动物体内可激发免疫应答,活化的免疫细胞可产生各种免疫分子,包括抗体、细胞因子和补体等,由活化的 B 淋巴细胞分化而来的浆细胞分泌抗体进入血液,从这种血液中分离出来的血清含有大量针对某种抗原的抗体,此种血清称为抗血清,或免疫血清(图 25-1)。抗血清中的抗体是针对抗原的多种表位,并由多个抗体形成细胞克隆分泌,故称为多克隆抗体。非可溶性形式或是加佐剂的抗原具有更强的免疫原性,最常用的佐剂是弗氏完全佐剂,可溶性抗原加佐剂能形成稳定的油包水乳剂。

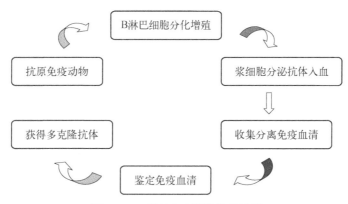

图 25-1　制备多克隆抗体的过程

【应用】

许多用于检测抗原的技术都是以抗原—抗体反应为基础,检测各种抗原的抗体可以从不同抗原免疫动物制备的抗血清获得。

【材料】

1. 小鼠 γ 球蛋白
2. 生理盐水
3. 弗氏完全佐剂和弗氏不完全佐剂
4. 双针头连接的两个注射器或研钵和研磨棒
5. 健康成年兔,体重 2~3 kg
6. 试管、离心机、水浴箱、冰箱等

【方法】

1. 将小鼠 γ 球蛋白 500 μg 溶解于 1 mL 生理盐水。

2. 逐滴加入 1 mL 弗氏完全佐剂中,用双针头连接的两个注射器或研钵和研磨棒混均,使加进的每滴抗原液成为乳剂。

3. 继续混匀,直至加进的全部抗原液成为乳剂,取 1 滴至冰水表面,若乳剂稳定,在冰水表面不会扩散。

4. 取 1 mL 乳剂在兔的颈背部和大腿分 5~6 个点肌肉或皮下注射。

5. 2 周后重复注射,若注射部位出现肉芽肿,第二次免疫可用弗氏不完全佐剂。

6. 再经 2 周后从兔耳动脉取血试测。

7. 将血置试管中,室温放置 1 h,使血液凝固收缩,再放 4℃中使血清释出。

8. 收集血清,以 2 000 r/min 离心 5 min 去除红细胞,用双向扩散试验检测效价。

【结果】

1. 如抗体效价低,可重复免疫 2~3 次。

2. 如抗体效价高,放血并收集血清。

3. 将血清置可长期保存的容器中,在 56℃ 作用 30 min,灭活不稳定的补体成分。

4. 抗血清保存在<-20℃或冷冻干燥后保存于<4℃。

【注意事项】

1. 制备纯化的、免疫原性强的抗原。

2. 选择健康、合适的动物,并细心饲养。

3. 制定可行的免疫方案,包括免疫的剂量、次数和途径等。

【思考题】

如果抗原免疫后产生的抗体效价低,其原因可能有哪些? 你如何解决此问题?

(田野平)

Exp. 25   Preparation of Polyclonal Antibody

【Principle】

Soluble antigens and granular antigens injected into an animal body can initiate immune responses. Activated immunocytes produce various immune molecules including antibodies, cytokines, complements and so on. Plasma cells derived from the activated B lymphocytes secrete antibodies into blood. Serum separated from this blood, which contains large quantities of antibodies against certain antigen, is called antiserum or immune serum (Fig.25 − 1). Antibodies in antiserum are against multiple epitopes of certain antigen and secreted by multiple clones of antibody forming cells, which are termed polyclonal antibody. Antigens are more immunogenic when presented in an insoluble form or with an adjuvant. The most commonly used adjuvant is Freund's complete adjuvant into which soluble antigen is combined as a stable water-in-oil emulsion.

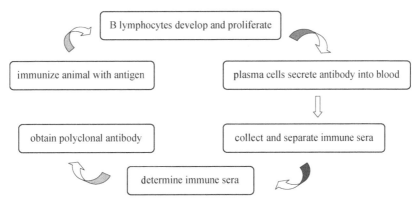

Fig.25 − 1   Process of polyclonal antibody preparation

【Application】

A number of immunologic techniques used in the detection of antigens are based on antigen-antibody interaction. Antibodies for detecting various antigens may be obtained from antisera prepared by immunizing the animals with different antigens.

【Materials】

1. Mouse γ globulin
2. Physiological saline
3. Freund's complete adjuvant and Freund's incomplete adjuvant
4. Double-hubbed needle attached two Luer-lock syringes or triturator and pestle
5. Healthy and adult rabbit, 2 − 3 kg
6. Test tubes, centrifuge, water bath, refrigerator, etc.

【Procedures】

1. Dissolve 500 μg of mouse γ globulin in 1 mL saline.

2. Add protein dropwise to 1 mL of Freund's complete adjuvant. Homogenize with triturator and pestle or double-hubbed needle attached two syringes until emulsion appears after adding each drop.

3. Continue homogenizing until a stable water-in-oil emulsion is obtained. Check this emulsion by gently placing one drop on the surface of a ice-water bath. If the emulsion is stable the drop will not disperse.

4. Inject approximately 1 mL of the emulsion intramuscularly or hypodermically at five or six different sites in the nuchal region and the thighs of the rabbit.

5. Repeat the injections two weeks later. If the granuloma ulcerates after the injection of antigen in Freund's complete adjuvant, it is suggested to take incomplete adjuvant in the second injection the following immunizations.

6. After two further weeks, test blood from the rabbit from the central ear artery.

7. Transfer the blood to a glass tube and allow it to clot at room temperature for 1 h. Loosen the clot from the tube to aid retraction. Store at 4℃ until serum is released.

8. Collect the released serum and centrifuge it at 2,000 r/min for 5 min to remove the erythrocytes.

Test the antiserum by double radial immunodiffusion test.

【Results】

1. Repeat injection 2－3 times if the antiserum titer is low.

2. If the antiserum titer is high enough, then bleed the rabbit and collect the serum.

3. Transfer the antiserum to the containers suitable for long-term storage and heat at 56℃ for 30 min to destroy the heat-labile components of complement.

4. The antiserum may be frozen at <−20℃ or freeze-dried and stored at <4℃.

【Precautions】

1. Prepare a purified antigen with strong immunogenicity.

2. Select healthy and suitable animals for immunization and feed them carefully.

3. Make a practicable immunization scheme including the dosage, the times and the way of immunization.

【Question】

What is the probable reason if the antibody titer is low after an antigen immunization? How do you solve this problem?

(Tian Yeping)

实验二十六　　多克隆抗体的纯化

【原理】

以抗原免疫动物来制备的抗血清是复杂的混合物，包括血清的全部成分。同抗原特异性结合的抗体主要是血清中的免疫球蛋白组分，因此需要分离和纯化。免疫球蛋白分子是一类蛋白质分子，与其他蛋白质一样，它有一定的等电点、溶解度、电荷电性及疏水性，可以用电泳、盐析沉淀或其他层析技术进行分离、纯化。目前，由于抗体免疫球蛋白的Fc 片段可以被蛋白 A、蛋白 G 结合，70%~80%的抗体纯化使用蛋白 A、蛋白 G 亲和层析。用蛋白 A、蛋白 G 一步亲和层析就可达到超过 95%的纯度。本实验介绍的是用蛋白 A 亲和层析纯化多克隆抗体的方法。该方法最为常用，也较其他方法简单和高效，能为常用的实验方法提供足够纯化的抗体，而且随着商品化的蛋白 A 基质的出现，能将任何来源的抗体纯化。蛋白 A 从金黄色葡萄球菌中获得，可与抗体重链的 Fc 片段相结合。如果将蛋白 A 与固相载体相连，如蛋白 A 交联琼脂糖凝胶（sepharose CL‑4B），这种填料可以成为分离和纯化抗体或抗体片段的重要工具。

【应用】

从抗血清中纯化多克隆抗体。

【材料】

1. 装有 2 mL 固相化的蛋白 A 的小型层析柱（如蛋白 A sepharose CL‑4B 亲和柱）
2. 透析袋（MWCO 10 000）
3. 结合缓冲液：0.1 mol/L Tris-HCl pH7.5 +0.15 mol/L NaCl
4. 洗脱缓冲液：0.1 mol/L Gly-HCl pH2.8 +0.15 mol/L NaCl
5. 中和缓冲液：1 mol/L Tris-HCl pH 8.0

【方法】

1. 样品预处理：样品在 4℃用结合缓冲液透析过夜，或将其与至少 1:1 稀释的结合缓冲液混合。
2. 准备蛋白 A 层析柱：至少用 10 mL 结合缓冲液，以 1 mL/min 的速度平衡洗涤柱中的 2 mL 亲和层析介质。
3. 加样：将透析后的样品加入亲和柱，一旦样品进入凝胶，用结合缓冲液洗柱（至少10 个柱的体积），直至 $A_{280\,nm}$小于 0.03。
4. 洗脱：用洗脱缓冲液洗脱所结合的抗体，分管收集（2 mL/管）。
5. 中和：收集过程中，每管立即加入 0.1 mL 中和缓冲液，以中和、洗脱所得的抗体液。

6. 保存：对含抗体的各管进行 PBS 透析,根据抗体的稳定性加入防腐剂(0.020 g/L 叠氮钠)后,可在 4℃或冷冻保存(图 26-1)。

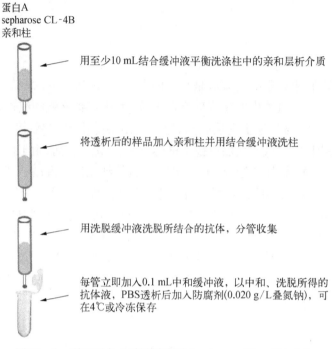

蛋白A
sepharose CL-4B
亲和柱

用至少 10 mL 结合缓冲液平衡洗涤柱中的亲和层析介质

将透析后的样品加入亲和柱并用结合缓冲液洗柱

用洗脱缓冲液洗脱所结合的抗体,分管收集

每管立即加入 0.1 mL 中和缓冲液,以中和、洗脱所得的抗体液,PBS 透析后加入防腐剂(0.020 g/L 叠氮钠),可在 4℃或冷冻保存

图 26-1 利用蛋白 A 琼脂糖凝胶(sepharose CL-4B)亲和柱纯化多克隆抗体的操作流程

【结果】

从含有血清所有成分的抗血清中分离、纯化多克隆抗体。

【注意事项】

1. 上样量由层析柱对特定免疫球蛋白的容量确定,2 mL 柱对于人 IgG 的容量约为 18 mg。

2. 柱上结合的抗体被洗脱的速度很快,通常在第一洗脱流分中。

3. 下列缓冲液也可用做结合缓冲液：含 0.15 mol/L NaCl 的 50 mmol/L 硼酸钠(pH8.0),或含 0.15 mol/L NaCl 的 0.1 mol/L 磷酸盐液(pH7.5)。高盐结合缓冲液(>1 mol/L NaCl)可能增加柱结合容量约 50%。

4. 对 pH 敏感的抗体,需用比较温和的洗脱液,如含 0.2 mol/L NaCl 的 0.1 mol/L Tris-乙酸 pH7.7,或 3 mol/L KCl,或 5.0 mol/L KI,或 3.5 mol/L MgCl$_2$。

5. 蛋白 A 亲和层析法还可用于：① 除去抗体溶液中 IgG,检测非 IgG 抗体(如 IgM)的生物活性或用于分离和纯化不同类型、不同亚类的抗体;② 除去木瓜蛋白酶或胃蛋白酶水解不同种类的抗体后的 Fc 片段;③ 回收或纯化免疫复合物。

6. 蛋白 G 和蛋白 A 的作用原理类似,都可以与抗体重链的 Fc 片段相结合,但在结合抗体的种类和强度上有所区别。

【思考题】

有哪些方法可用于多克隆抗体的纯化？各有哪些优缺点？

（龚文容）

Exp. 26　Purification of Polyclonal Antibody

【Principle】

An antiserum prepared by immunizing animals with antigen is a complex mixture, including all components of the serum. Antibodies specifically binding to the antigen are mainly the immunoglobulin components in the serum and therefore need to be separated and purified. Immunoglobulin molecules are a class of protein molecules. Like other proteins, they have a certain isoelectric point, solubility, charge and hydrophobicity, which can be separated and purified by electrophoretic, salting precipitation or other chromatography techniques. Currently, since the Fc fragment of the antibody immunoglobulin can be bound by protein A/G, about 70% – 80% antibodies Igs can be purified by using protein A /G affinity chromatography. The purity can reach over 95% by protein A or protein G affinity chromatography. The method of purification of polyclonal antibody by protein A affinity chromatography is introduced in this experiment. The method is most commonly used, and is simple and efficient compared with other methods. It can provide enough purified antibodies for common experimental methods, and antibodies can be purified from any source with the emergence of commercialized protein A matrix. Protein A is obtained from *Staphylococcus aureus* and can bind the Fc fragment of antibody heavy chain. If protein A is linked to a solid phase carrier, such as protein A crosslinked agarose gel (Sepharose CL−4B), this kind of filler can be used as an important tool for the separation and purification of antibody or antibody fragments.

【Application】

Purify polyclonal antibody from antiserum.

【Materials】

1. Small chromatographic columns containing 2 mL solid phase protein A (e. g. protein A Sepharose CL−4B affinity column)
2. Dialysis membranes (MWCO 10,000)
3. Binding buffer: 0. 1 mol/L Tris-HCl pH7. 5 +0. 15 mol/L NaCl
4. Elution buffer: 0. 1 mol/L Gly-HCl pH2. 8+0. 15 mol/L NaCl
5. Neutralizing buffer: 1 mol/L Tris-HCl pH 8

【Procedures】

1. Speciman pretreatment: samples were dialysated overnight with binding buffer at 4℃ or diluted with binding buffer at least 1 : 1.

2. Preparation of protein A chromatographic column: the 2 mL affinity chromatographic medium in the washing column is balanced with at least 10 mL binding buffer at 1 mL/min speed.

3. Sample loading into the colum: after dialysis, load samples to the affinity column. Once the sample entered into the gel, wash the column with binding buffer (at least 10 times colum volume) until the value of A_{280} nm was less than 0.03.

4. Elution: Elute the antibodies with elution buffer and collect (2 mL/tube).

5. Neutralization: during the collection process, add 0.1 mL neutralization buffer each tube to neutralize the eluted antibody solution.

6. Preservation: tubes containing antibodies are subjected to PBS dialysis, followed by the addition of preservatives (0.020 g/L azide sodium) according to the stability of the antibody, then store them at 4℃ or cryopreserved(Fig.26 - 1).

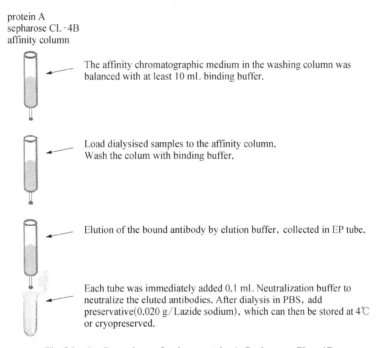

protein A
sepharose CL-4B
affinity column

The affinity chromatographic medium in the washing column was balanced with at least 10 mL binding buffer.

Load dialysised samples to the affinity column.
Wash the colum with binding buffer.

Elution of the bound antibody by elution buffer, collected in EP tube.

Each tube was immediately added 0.1 mL Neutralization buffer to neutralize the eluted antibodies. After dialysis in PBS, add preservative(0.020 g/Lazide sodium), which can then be stored at 4℃ or cryopreserved.

Fig.26 - 1　Procedure of using protein A Sepharose CL - 4B
affinity column to purify polyclonal antibody

【Results】

Polyclonal antibody can be separated and purified from antiserum which includes all components of the serum.

【Precautions】

1. The amount of the loading sample is determined by the capacity of the column to the immunoglobulin. The capacity of the 2 mL column for human IgG is about 18 mg.

2. The antibody binding to the column is eluted rapidly, usually in the first eluent.

3. The following buffer can also be used as binding buffer: 50 mmol/L sodium borate (pH8.0) containing 0.15 mol/L NaCl, or 0.1 mol/L phosphate solution (pH7.5) containing 0.15 mol/L NaCl. High salt binding buffer (>1 mol/L NaCl) may increase the total column binding capacity by about 50%.

4. For pH sensitive antibodies, a relatively mild eluent should be used, such as 0.1 mol/L Tris-acetate pH7.7 containing 0.2 mol/L NaCl or 3 mol/L KCl or 5.0 mol/L KI or 3.5 mol/L $MgCl_2$.

5. Protein A affinity chromatography can also be used for following purpose: ① to remove IgG in the antibody solution, to detect the biological activity of non IgG antibodies (such as IgM) or to separate and purify different types, subclass antibodies; ② to remove Fc segments after papain or pepsin hydrolysate of different types of antibodies; ③ to recover or purify immune complex.

6. The principle of protein G and protein A for purify Ig (antibody) is similar, both can bind the Fc fragment of the antibody heavy chain, but the binding is different in type and intensity of antibodies.

【Question】

What are the methods for purifying polyclonal antibodies, and what are the advantages and disadvantages?

(Gong Wenrong)

实验二十七　单克隆抗体制备

【原理】

被抗原致敏的 B 淋巴细胞能分泌特异性抗体,但不能在体外长期存活。B 细胞骨髓瘤可在体外长期存活并大量繁殖,但不能分泌抗体。应用聚乙二醇使小鼠骨髓瘤细胞与来自经抗原免疫的同系小鼠脾细胞(含有产生抗体的 B 淋巴细胞)融合,再用选择培养液进行选择培养。选择培养液含有次黄嘌呤(H)、氨基蝶呤(A)和胸腺嘧啶核苷(T),即 HAT 培养液。氨基蝶呤是叶酸拮抗物,能阻断 DNA 合成的主要途径。次黄嘌呤和胸腺嘧啶核苷是合成 DNA 的原料。当合成 DNA 的主要途径受阻时,正常细胞可通过次黄嘌呤鸟嘌呤磷酸核糖转移酶(HGPRT)或胸腺嘧啶核苷激酶(TK),利用次黄嘌呤和胸腺嘧啶核苷由旁路途径(挽救途径)合成 DNA 而生存。但自相融合或未融合的骨髓瘤细胞由于缺乏 HGPRT 或 TK,无法由旁路途径合成 DNA 而死亡。自相融合或未融合的 B 淋巴细胞虽具有合成 DNA 旁路途径的酶,但在体外培养中存活常不超过 2 周。唯独杂交瘤细胞因具有骨髓瘤细胞长期生存的特点,又获得了 B 淋巴细胞的酶和产生特异性抗体的能力,得以在 HAT 培养液中生存并分泌抗体,再经反复的克隆化培养,可获得由一个杂交瘤细胞繁衍而来的单克隆杂交瘤细胞,所产生的抗体称为单克隆抗体(图 27 - 1)。

【应用】

单克隆抗体作为一种工具,广泛地应用于临床实验诊断和基础医学研究,如病原体的鉴定、血清中各种蛋白质的检测及细胞表面分子的测定。

【材料】

1. RPMI - 1640 完全培养液(含 10% 新生小牛血清)
2. RPMI - 1640 无血清培养液
3. 50% 聚乙二醇(PEG),MW 1 500,50% m/V
4. HAT 培养液
5. 无 Ca^{2+}、Mg^{2+} Hank's 液
6. 降植烷
7. 小鼠骨髓瘤细胞(Sp2/0 细胞系)
8. 抗原免疫的 BALB/c 小鼠
9. 96 孔培养板
10. 塑料圆锥底离心管(50 mL)
11. 培养瓶(10 mL)和培养皿
12. 不锈钢网(200 目)
13. 吸管、滴管、剪刀、镊子、水浴箱、CO_2 孵箱等

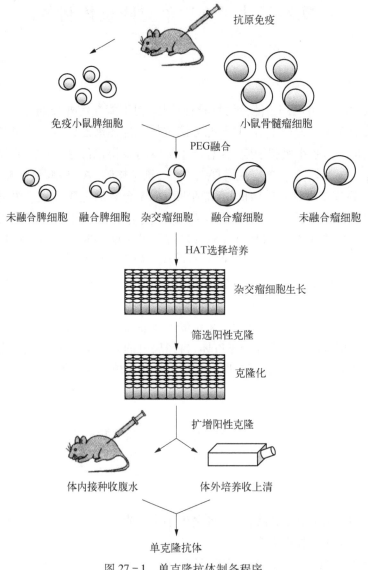

抗原免疫

免疫小鼠脾细胞　　　　　小鼠骨髓瘤细胞

PEG融合

未融合脾细胞　融合脾细胞　杂交瘤细胞　融合瘤细胞　未融合瘤细胞

HAT选择培养

杂交瘤细胞生长

筛选阳性克隆

克隆化

扩增阳性克隆

体内接种收腹水　　　　体外培养收上清

单克隆抗体

图 27-1　单克隆抗体制备程序

【方法】

1. 免疫小鼠和骨髓瘤细胞准备:

(1) 用需要制备相应单克隆抗体的抗原免疫小鼠。

(2) 将小鼠骨髓瘤细胞用 RPMI-1640 完全培养液在培养瓶中进行扩大培养。

(3) 选择生长旺盛、活力>95%的骨髓瘤细胞,收集于 50 mL 圆锥底离心管中,以 1 000 r/min 离心 15 min。

(4) 弃上清,沉淀细胞用 RPMI-1640 无血清培养液洗涤 2 次,以 1 000 r/min 离心 15 min。

（5）用 RPMI‐1640 无血清培养液重悬末次沉淀细胞，计数活细胞，配成 1×10^6 个/mL，以备融合用。

2. 巨噬细胞饲养层的制备：

（1）将 5 mL 无 Ca^{2+}、Mg^{2+} Hank's 液注入正常小鼠腹腔，抽出含腹腔巨噬细胞的液体，置 50 mL 圆锥底离心管中，此过程反复进行 2~3 次。

（2）用无 Ca^{2+}、Mg^{2+} Hank's 液洗涤细胞 1 次，以 1 000 r/min 离心 10 min。

（3）用培养液重悬沉淀细胞，计数并调节细胞浓度至 2×10^5 个/mL。

（4）加入 96 孔培养板，每孔 100 μL。

（5）置 37℃、5% CO_2 孵箱培养，于次日使用。

3. 免疫小鼠脾细胞悬液的制备：

（1）无菌条件下取免疫小鼠脾脏，置培养皿中的 200 目不锈钢网上。

（2）加少量 RPMI‐1640 无血清培养液，用注射器内芯平端将脾脏轻轻压过钢网，取出钢网，用滴管轻轻吹吸分散细胞。

（3）以 RPMI‐1640 无血清培养液洗涤 1 次，以 1 000 r/min 离心 10 min。

（4）沉淀细胞重悬于 5 mL RPMI‐1640 无血清培养液。计数淋巴细胞，以备融合用。

4. 细胞融合：

（1）取制备好的骨髓瘤细胞与脾淋巴细胞，以 1∶5~1∶10 比例在 50 mL 试管中混合，以 1 000 r/min 离心 10 min。

（2）弃净上清，轻轻叩松留存管内的沉淀细胞。

（3）将细胞、50%PEG 及 RPMI‐1640 无血清培养液均置于 37℃ 水浴箱中预温。

（4）将 50% PEG 0.8 mL 于 1 min 内逐滴加入细胞沉淀中，37℃ 水浴箱中静置 1 min。

（5）逐渐加入预温的无血清 RPMI‐1640 培养液 30~40 mL，轻轻摇动试管，在 5 min 内加完。此时要慢加，因 PEG 作用后，细胞对机械损伤敏感。

（6）在室温中以 1 000 r/min 离心 10 min。

（7）弃上清，沉淀细胞用 10 mL 含 10%小牛血清的 HAT 培养液重新悬浮。

（8）滴加于预先铺有饲养细胞的 96 孔培养板中，每孔加 100 μL。

（9）将培养板置 37℃、5% CO_2 孵箱中培养。

5. 杂交瘤细胞的克隆化（有限稀释法）：在显微镜下观察到杂交瘤细胞开始成簇生长，应及时筛选产生抗体的阳性孔。筛选大量培养板孔中的上清，以鉴定出具有所需特性的抗体，这需要简便的技术。有几种技术适合筛选抗体，如酶联免疫法就是最常用的检测可溶性分子的方法。一旦筛选到有抗体活性的阳性孔，尽快进行克隆化和重测，有限稀释法是进行杂交瘤细胞克隆化的主要方法。

（1）于 96 孔平底微量培养板制备巨噬细胞饲养层，用一块或半块板作一个阳性孔杂交瘤细胞的克隆化。

（2）收集并计数各阳性孔中的细胞。

（3）分别制备 20 个/mL、10 个/mL、5 个/mL 的细胞悬液。

（4）分别加入 96 孔培养板，每孔 100 μL。

（5）培养板置 37℃、5% CO_2 孵箱中培养。1~2 周后可观察到克隆生长。

（6）检测上清中抗体,将阳性孔中杂交瘤细胞再次选出培养并作克隆化。

6. 杂交瘤细胞系的建立与维持：杂交瘤细胞系在固定的培养瓶或旋转的培养罐中生长到稳定期,可以产生 1 μg/mL 抗体蛋白。将杂交瘤细胞系分别注入组织相容性的小鼠腹腔,可以产生大量的单克隆抗体($5 \sim 20$ mg/mL)。

（1）每只小鼠腹腔内注射 0.5 mL 降植烷。

（2）7 天后于小鼠腹腔内注射 1×10^6 个杂交瘤细胞,$2 \sim 3$ 周大多数可产生实体瘤和腹水。

（3）用注射器抽出腹水,在 4℃ 以 2 000 r/min 离心 15 min,腹水冻存于$-70℃$。

（4）小鼠存活期间可重复进行以上第 3 步。

【结果】

1. 杂交瘤细胞加冻存液置于冻存管,保存于液氮中。
2. 检定杂交瘤细胞系的染色体数。
3. 鉴定单克隆抗体对抗原的特异性。
4. 鉴定单克隆抗体免疫球蛋白类型和亚类。
5. 测定单克隆抗体的效价。
6. 测定单克隆抗体的亲和力。

【注意事项】

1. 为了保持骨髓瘤细胞系 HGPRT 和 TK 缺陷,可将细胞每 $3 \sim 6$ 个月在含有 8 -氮鸟嘌呤或 6 -巯基鸟嘌呤(2×10^{-5} mol/L)的培养液中进行培养,以去除对 HAT 抵抗的回复变异细胞。

2. 用于融合的骨髓瘤细胞活力应在 95% 以上。

3. 加入培养液中的新生小牛血清应预先进行筛选,以利于单个克隆细胞的生长。

4. 氨基蝶呤具有高度毒性,且为强致癌剂。氨基蝶呤必须避光。

5. 选择培养后,勿将杂交瘤细胞从 HAT 培养液直接转换到正常培养液,因为残留的氨基蝶呤能阻止 DNA 合成的恢复,而是让细胞在 RPMI -1640 完全培养液中继续培养 $3 \sim 5$ 天后再转换正常培养液。

6. 必须对杂交瘤细胞系反复克隆化以保证其均一性。

7. 实验操作需在无菌条件下进行。

【思考题】

1. 单克隆抗体与多克隆抗体在制备和性质方面的主要差别是什么？

2. 骨髓瘤细胞与脾细胞融合后未筛选到阳性杂交瘤细胞克隆,其可能的原因有哪些？

（田野平）

Exp. 27　Preparation of Monoclonal Antibody

【Principle】

B lymphocytes sensitized by an antigen can secrete the specific antibodies but are unable to surive *in vitro* for a long time. The immortal B-cell myeloma can grow and reproduce generously *in vitro* but not secrete its own antibody. Splenocytes containing antibody-producing B lymphocytes, prepared from the antigen immunized mice, are induced to fuse with murine myeloma cells from the same strain using polyethylene glycol (PEG) and then cultured in a selective medium. The selective medium contains hypoxanthine, aminopterin and thymidine (HAT medium). Aminopterin is an antagonist of folic acid and blocks the main pathway of DNA synthesis. Hypoxanthine and thymidine are the pre-formed bases for DNA synthesis. When the main pathway of DNA synthesis is blocked, the normal cells are able to synthesize DNA by hypoxanthine-guanine-phosphoribosyl transferase (HGPRT) or thymidine kinase (TK) via the bypass pathway, the so-called salvage pathway, using hypoxanthine and thymidine to grow in this medium. Un-fused myeloma cells or self-fused myeloma cells die in HAT medium, as they are deficient in the HGPRT or TK and cannot utilize hypoxanthine and thymidine to synthesize DNA via the salvage pathway. Although un-fused B lymphocytes or self-fused B lymphocytes have the enzymes to synthesize DNA via the bypass pathway, they die *in vitro* culture naturally within 2 weeks. Only the hybridoma cells produced by the fusion between myeloma cells and B lymphocytes survive and secrete antibodies in HAT medium because they obtain the potential immortality provided by myeloma cells and the enzymes as well as the ability generating the specific antibodies from B lymphocytes. Then the hybridoma cells are cloned repeatedly. Antibody secreted by a clone of cells derived from a single hybridoma cell is called monoclonal antibody (Fig.27－1).

【Application】

Monoclonal antibody as a tool has the broad application ranges in clinical experimental diagnosis and basic medicine research, for example pathogen identification, various proteins assay in serum, detection of molecules on cell surface and so on.

【Materials】

1. Complete RPMI－1640 medium (supplemented with 10% newborn calf serum)
2. Serum-free RPMI－1640 medium
3. Polyethylene glycol (PEG), MW1500, 50% *m/V*
4. HAT medium

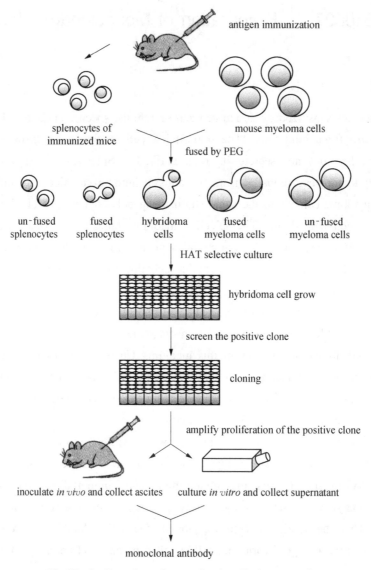

Fig.27 - 1　Procedure of monoclonal antibody preparation

5. Ca^{2+}-and Mg^{2+}-free Hank's balanced salt solution

6. Pristane

7. Mouse myeloma cells (Sp2/0 cell line)

8. BALB/c mice immunized with required antigen

9. Culture plate, 96 micro-wells, flat bottom

10. Plastic conical centrifuge tubes, 50 mL, sterile

11. Sterilized culture dishes and culture flasks (10 mL culture volume)

12. Sterilized stainless steel screen (200-mesh)

13. Pipettes, droppers, scissors, forceps, water bath, incubator, etc.

〔Procedures〕

1. Preparation of immunized mice and myeloma cells:

(1) Immunize mice with the antigens.

(2) Culture myeloma cells with complete RPMI – 1640 medium in culture flask.

(3) Select the exuberant myeloma cells with >95% viability, collect them into a 50 mL conical centrifuge tube and centrifuge at 1,000 r/min for 15 min.

(4) Remove the supernatant and wash the cells twice by centrifugation at 2,000 r/min for 15 min with serum-free RPMI – 1640 medium.

(5) Re-suspend the final pellet in serum-free RPMI – 1640 medium, count the number of viable cells and adjust to 1×10^6 cells/mL for fusion use.

2. Preparation of macrophage feeder layers:

(1) Inject 5 mL of Ca^{2+}-and Mg^{2+}-free Hank's solution into a normal mouse peritoneal cavity, take out the liquid containing peritoneal macrophages and pour them into a 50 mL conical centrifuge tube. Repeat this process 2 – 3 times.

(2) Wash the cells once in Ca^{2+}-and Mg^{2+}-free Hank's solution by centrifugation at 1,000 r/min for 10 min.

(3) Re-suspend the final pellet in medium, count and adjust the cells to 2×10^5/mL.

(4) Dispense 100 μL aliquots into each well of the 96 well micro-culture plate.

(5) Incubate in a humid 37℃ incubator gassed with 5% CO_2 in air and use them next day.

3. Preparation of splenocyte suspension of the immunized mice:

(1) Remove the immunized mouse spleen and put it on a stainless steel 200-mesh strainer in a dish.

(2) Add 1 mL serum-free RPMI – 1640 medium to the dish, push the spleen slightly through the screen with the flat top surface of a syringe core, take out the screen and disperse the cells by slightly sucking splenocyte suspensions in and out of a dropper.

(3) Wash splenocytes once by centrifugation at 1,000 r/min for 10 min.

(4) Re-suspend the cell pellet in 5 mL of serum-free RPMI – 1640 medium. Count the number of viable lymphocytes and reserve them for fusion.

4. Cell fusion:

(1) Mix myeloma cells with splenocytes at 1 : 5 – 1 : 10 ratio in a 50 mL conical tube and centrifuge at 1,000 r/min for 10 min.

(2) Decant the supernatant carefully and completely. Mix cell pellet by gently tapping the tube.

(3) Allow the cells, PEG solution and serum-free RPMI – 1640 medium to equilibrate to 37℃ in a water bath.

(4) Add 0.8 mL of PEG to re-suspended cells within 1 min, rock gently and incubate

cells at 37℃ for 1 min.

(5) Gradually add 30 – 40 mL of serum-free medium over 5 min with gentle shaking. Dilution must be done slowly as the cells are very sensitive to mechanical damage in the PEG solution.

(6) Centrifuge at 1,000 r/min for 10 min at room temperature.

(7) Remove the supernatant and re-suspend the cell pellet in 10 mL of HAT selective medium containing 10% new born calf serum.

(8) Dispense 100 μL aliquots of cell suspension into each well of the 96-well culture plate laid with feeder cells in advance.

(9) Place all the plates in a humid 37℃ incubator gassed with 5% CO_2.

5. Cloning by limiting dilution: the initial screen of the positive wells for antibody activity should be carried out as soon as clustered growth of hybridoma cells is observed under the microscope. Technically simple and convenient assay are required so that a large number of supernatants can be screened to identify the wells containing the antibody with the required properties. Several techniques are preferable for screening antibody activity, for example enzyme-inked immunoassay is the most commen technique to detect soluble molecules. Once antibody activity has been detected in any particular well, it is essential to clone and re-test the cells as soon as possible. Limiting dilution is the main method for cloning the hybridoma cells secreting antibody.

(1) Prepare macrophage feeder layers in 96-well, flat-bottom micro-culture plates; allow one or half plate for hybridoma cells in each positive well to be cloned.

(2) Harvest and count the cells of each positive well.

(3) Prepare cell suspensions at 20, 10 and 5 cells/mL respectively.

(4) Add 100 μL aliquots of the cells/mL suspension to each of 96 wells respectively.

(5) Incubate the plates in a humid 37℃ incubator gassed with 5% CO_2 in air. Colonies should be visible after 1 – 2 weeks.

(6) Test supernatants for antibody activity and select positive wells for culture and cloning again.

6. Initiation and maintenance of hybridoma cell lines: when hybridoma cell lines are allowed to grow up to stationary phase in static flasks or spinner culture vessels, they can produce up to 1 μg/mL of antibody protein. Large amounts of monoclonal antibodies (5 – 20 mg/mL) may be prepared by injecting these hybridoma cell lines into histocompatible mice respectively.

(1) Inject 0.5 mL pristine into the peritoneal cavity of each mouse.

(2) After 7 days, inject 10^6 hybridoma cells i. p. into each mouse. Most hybridoma lines will produce solid tumors or ascites within 2 – 3 weeks.

(3) Use a syringe to drain off the ascitic fluid. Clarify the ascitic fluid by centrifugation (2,000 r/min for 15 min at 4℃). The fluid should be stored at −70℃.

(4) Repeat step 3 during the lifetime of the mice.

【Results】

1. Add hybridoma cells with cold storage medium to the vials and store in liquid nitrogen.

2. Check the chromosome numbers of hybridoma cell line.

3. Test the specificity of the antibody.

4. Identify class and subclass of immunoglobulin of the monoclonal antibody.

5. Determine the titre of monoclonal antibody.

6. Determine the affinity of monoclonal antibody.

【Precautions】

1. Keep the myeloma cell line in HGPRT and TK deficiency, eliminate revertants to HAT resistance by culturing the myeloma cell lines in medium containing 8-azaguanine or 6-thioguanine (2×10^{-5} mol/L) every 3 – 6 months.

2. The viability of myeloma cell used for fusion should be above 95%.

3. New born calf serum supplemented in culture medium should be selected in advance to benefit single clone growth of the cells.

4. Aminopterin is highly toxic and a potent carcinogen. Aminopterin must be protected from light.

5. After the selection phase is complete, do not transfer the hybridoma cells directly from HAT medium to normal culture medium as sufficient aminopterin may be carried over to prevent a resumption of DNA synthesis. Instead, culture the cells in complete RPMI – 1640 medium for 3 – 5 days before transferring to normal culture medium.

6. Cloning must be repeated to ensure the homogeneity of hybridoma cell line.

7. The experimental operation should be proceeded in an aseptic condition.

【Questions】

1. What are the main differences between monoclonal antibody and polyclonal antibody in the preparation and the property?

2. What are the probable reasons if the positive clone of hybridoma cells is not screened out after the fusion of myeloma cells and splenocytes?

(Tian Yeping)

实验二十八　　单链抗体（scFv）的构建

【原理】

单链抗体（scFv）是一种新型重组蛋白,是将抗体重链（V_H）可变区和轻链（V_L）可变区片段用一条弹性短肽连接而成的小分子抗体片段。scFv 主要是从杂交瘤细胞构建而成。再从杂交瘤细胞中提取含抗体 V_H、V_L 可变区的 mRNA,经反转录聚合酶链反应将 mRNA 反转录成 cDNA;PCR 分别扩增 V_H、V_L 可变区的 cDNA,并通过重叠 PCR 由连接序列（Gly4Ser）3 将 2 段序列连接成一条 cDNA,再克隆到原核或真核表达载体中,即可产生目的 scFv。

【应用】

scFv 具有分子量小、穿透性强等特点,在免疫分析、疾病诊断和治疗中应用广泛。scFv 作为靶向载体连接放射性核素、生物素和酶形成融合蛋白,借助抗原抗体相反应的特异性进行免疫显像诊断,具有较高的特异性和敏感性。scFv 也可以连接放射性核素、免疫毒素和药物,将其靶向运输到病灶部位,不仅能使病灶部位达到较高的药物浓度,更好地发挥药效,而且减少药物对正常组织的毒副作用,因而具有广泛的应用前景。本实验以构建人源性 anti-TNF－α 为例,阐述 scFv 的构建。

【材料】

1. 抗 TNF－α 杂交瘤细胞株
2. 大肠杆菌 BL21（DE3）株、表达载体 pGEX－4T－1
3. 引物
4. 主要试剂:胎牛血清、杂交瘤细胞培养基、RNA 提取试剂、反转录 PCR 试剂、高保真 PCR 试剂、*Sal*I 内切酶、*Not*I 内切酶、T4 DNA 连接酶和 IPTG 等

【方法】

1. 制备抗 TNF－α 杂交瘤细胞株的总 cDNA:

（1）复苏、培养冻存抗 TNF－α 杂交瘤细胞株。

（2）收获 1×10^6 个细胞株,使用 RNA 提取试剂盒提取细胞 mRNA,溶于 20 μL 无酶水。

（3）以总 mRNA 为模板,转录成总 cDNA,反应体系、程序如下:

Oligo（dT）	2 μL
RNA	X μL（≤1 μg）
无酶 H_2O	$23 - X$ μL

70℃ 10 min,4℃ 10 min 后加入下列成分

5×RT 缓冲液	8 μL
dNTP 混合液(10 mmol/L)	4 μL
Ace	2 μL
RNase 抑制剂(10 U/μL)	1 μL
总计	40 μL

42℃ 1 h,94℃ 10 min,25℃ 2 min

(4) cDNA 分装,-20℃冻存。

2. 扩增抗 TNF-α 的 V_H 和 V_L 的 cDNA:

(1) 设计、合成针对 V_H 和 V_L 的引物。根据 Ig 可变区基因序列特点,以及已经发表的小鼠 V_H 和 V_L 基因序列,分别设计对应不同亚类 Ig 骨架 FR1 和 FR4 序列的通用引物。其序列如下:

V_H 5′端引物(F1): 5′-CAGTGGATAGACCGATGGGGG-3′

V_H 3′端引物(R1): 5′-ATGATGGTGTTAAGTCCTTCTGTA-3′

V_L 5′端引物(F2): 5′-ATGGAGACAGACACACTCCTGCTAT-3′

V_L 3′端引物(R2): 5′-GGATACAGTTGGTGCAGCATCAGCCCGT-3′

(2) 以总 cDNA 为模板,分别以 F1、R1 和 F2、R2 为引物,扩增目的抗体的 V_H 和 V_L 的 cDNA,反应体系、程序如下:

10×PCR 缓冲液	5 μL
2 mmol/L dNTP	5 μL
25 mmol/L MgSO$_4$	3 μL
F1/F2	1 μL
R1/R2	1 μL
cDNA	1 μL(~200 ng)
KOD-Plus-Neo(高保真 *Taq* DNA 聚合酶)	1 μL
ddH$_2$O	33 μL
总计	50 μL

94℃ 5 min, 30 次循环: 94℃ 15 s、56℃ 15 s、72℃ 45 s,72℃ 10 min

(3) PCR 产物 2%琼脂凝胶电泳,并回收 480 bp 大小的目的片段,溶于 30 μL ddH$_2$O。

(4) PCR 产物测序,通过与 Pubmed 和 IMGT 等数据库比较 DNA 序列和对应的蛋白质(Ig)序列,序列对比正确后-20℃冻存

3. 重叠 PCR 构建 V_H-连接片段-V_L:

(1) 利用重叠 PCR 把 V_H 和 V_L 2 条 DNA 链通过连接片段连接成一条链,并且为便于插入表达载体,在 V_H 的正向引物和 V_L 的反向引物 5′端分别引入酶切位点,引物如下:

V_H 5′端引物(F3): 5′-ATT<u>GCGGCCGC</u>TTATGGGGGTGTTGGGC-3′(下划线代表 *Sal*I)

V_H 3′端引物(R3): 5′-<u>ACTACCGCCTCCACCACTACCGCCTCCACCACTACCGC</u>
<u>CTCCACC</u>GAGGTGCAGCTTCAGGAG-3′(下划线代表 Gly4Ser)3

V_L 5′端引物(F4): 5′-<u>GGGTGGAGGCGGTAGTGGTGGAGGCGGTAGTGGTGGA</u>
<u>GGCGGTAGT</u>CCGTTTGATCTCCAGCTT-3′(下划线代表 Gly4Ser)3

$V_L 3'$ 端引物(R4): $5' -$ ATT<u>GTCGAC</u>TCGAGTCACATTCTCAGCTC $-3'$(下划线代表 *Not*I)

(2) 分别以回收 V_H 和 V_L 的 PCR 产物为模板,加入上述引物,扩增插入了酶切位点和连接片段序列的 V_H 和 V_L,反应体系、程序如下:

10×PCR 缓冲液	5 μL
2 mmol/L dNTP	5 μL
25 mmol/L MgSO₄	3 μL
F3/F4	1 μL
R3/R4	1 μL
cDNA	1 μL(~200 ng)
KOD-Plus-Neo(高保真 *Taq* DNA 聚合酶)	1 μL
ddH₂O	33 μL
总计	50 μL

94℃ 5 min, 30 次循环: 94℃ 15 s、56℃ 15 s、72℃ 60 s,72℃ 10 min

(3) PCR 产物 2% 琼脂凝胶电泳,并回收 550 bp 大小的目的片段,溶于 30 μL ddH₂O。

(4) 以回收 PCR 产物为模板,以 $V_H 5'$ 端引物(F3)和 $V_L 3'$ 端引物(R4)为引物,扩增插入了酶切位点的 $V_H - V_L$ 序列反应体系、程序如下:

10×PCR 缓冲液	5 μL
2 mmol/L dNTP	5 μL
25 mmol/L MgSO₄	3 μL
F3	1 μL
R4	1 μL
cDNA	1 μL(~200 ng)
KOD-Plus-Neo(高保真 Taq DNA 聚合酶)	1 μL
ddH₂O	33 μL
总计	50 μL

94℃ 5 min, 30 循环: 94℃ 15 s、56℃ 15 s、72℃ 90 s,72℃ 10 min

(5) PCR 产物 1.5% 琼脂凝胶电泳,并回收 1 100 bp 大小的目的片段,溶于 30 μL ddH₂O,分装、−20℃ 冻存。

4. 构建 $V_H - V_L$ 原核表达质粒:

(1) 分别以 *Sal*I 和 *Not*I 双酶切原核表达载体 pGEX−4T−1 和回收 PCR 产物(V_H−连接片段−V_L),酶切体系如下:

10×Cut Smart 缓冲液	2 μL
*Sal*I	1 μL
*Not*I	1 μL
pGEX−4T−1/V_H−连接片段−V_L	X μL (≤1 μg)
ddH₂O	$20 - X$ μL
总计	20 μL

37℃水浴 2 h

（2）酶切体系 1%琼脂凝胶电泳,并回收酶切产物。

（3）T4 DNA 连接酶连接回收的酶切产物,反应体系如下:

10×T4 DNA 连接酶　Buffer	2 μL
pGEX-4T-1	1 μL
V_H - V_L	3 μL
T4	1 μL
ddH_2O	13 μL
总计	20 μL

16℃水浴 16 h

（4）连接体系转化大肠杆菌 BL21(DE3)株,因为表达载体 pGEX-4T-1 含氨苄西林抗性基因,连接成功的质粒在含氨苄西林的琼脂平皿中可以生长,而没连接成功的载体不能在抗性平皿上生长,挑选阳性克隆。

（5）培养阳性克隆菌株,提取质粒,SalⅠ 和 NotⅠ 双酶切鉴定,阳性克隆出现 4 900 bp 和 1 100 bp 2 条目的条带。

（6）鉴定正确的克隆株扩大培养,在菌液 OD 值为 0.6~0.8 时加入 IPTG,诱导目的蛋白在细菌中表达,通过 GST 标签纯化 V_H -连接片段- V_L,即可以收获抗 TNF-α 单链抗体。

【结果】

1. scFv 成功从杂交瘤细胞株中克隆出来,并插入原核表达载体 pGEX-4T-1,构建了抗 TNF-α 的 scFv(图 28-1)。

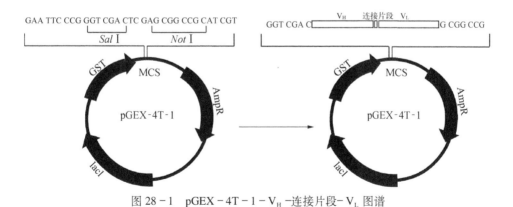

图 28-1　pGEX-4T-1-V_H-连接片段-V_L 图谱

2. 阳性克隆的 SalⅠ 和 NotⅠ 双酶切鉴定,阳性克隆出现 4 900 bp 和 1 100 bp 2 条目的条带。

3. 诱导目的蛋白表达,收获抗 TNF-α 单链抗体

【注意事项】

1. 引物设计:根据免疫球蛋白家族最好设计多组引物,以便能扩增出大多数单克隆

抗体的 V_H 和 V_L 基因。

2. ScFv 有 2 种形式: V_H 的 C 端与 V_L 的 N 端连接,也可以 V_L 的 C 端与 V_H 的 N 端连接。

3. 构建质粒: 可以通过重叠 PCR 的产物 V_H-连接片段-V_L 与 T 载体连接后再把目的片段插入表达载体。

【思考题】

1. 连接片段具有哪些特点?

2. 怎样判定抗 TNF-α scFv 的质量?

3. 连接片段可以插入哪些表达载体? 不同表达载体各具有哪些优缺点?

(李平飞　郝雪艳)

Exp. 28　　Generation of scFv

【Principle】

A single-chain fragment variable (scFv) is a fusion protein of the variable regions of the heavy (V_H) and light chains (V_L) of immunoglobulins, connected with a short linker peptide. scFv has been constructed mainly from hybridoma spleen cells from immunize. The mRNA containing the V_H and V_L variable regions of the antibody were extracted from the hybridoma cells, and the mRNA were reverse transcribed into cDNA by reverse transcription polymerase chain reaction; PCR amplified the cDNA of the heavy chain and light chain variable regions, then linking two sequences into one cDNA by the linker sequence (Gly4Ser)3, and then clones into a prokaryotic or eukaryotic expression vector to produce scFv.

【Application】

scFv is widely used in immunoassays, disease diagnosis and treatment because of relatively low molecular weight and strong penetrability. scFv is applied to immunoimaging with high specificity and sensitivity by connecting the radionuclide, biotin or enzyme. scFv is also linked to radionuclides, immunotoxins or drugs, and then transported to the lesion. scFv not only increases drug concentration, but reduces the side effects of the drug, thus has a wide range of applications. Here, construction of anti-TNF$-\alpha$ scFv is used as an example.

【Materials】

1. Anti-TNF$-\alpha$ hybridoma cell line
2. *E. coli* BL21 (DE3) strain, prokaryotic expression vector pGEX$-4T-1$
3. Primers
4. Reagents: fetal bovine serum, hybridoma cell culture medium, RNA extraction reagent, reverse transcription PCR reagent, PCR reagent, restriction endonucleases *Sal*I and *Not*I, T4 DNA ligase, IPTG, etc.

【Procedures】

1. Preparation of total cDNA of anti-TNF$-\alpha$ hybridoma cell lines:

(1) Resuscitate and culture anti-TNF$-\alpha$ hybridoma cell lines.

(2) Harvest 1×10^6 cells. Total RNA of the cells is extracted by RNA extraction kit, then dissolved in 20 μL of nuclease-free water.

(3) Total mRNA as a template is transcribed as total cDNA. The following reagents are

used for reverse transcription cDNA：

Oligo（dT）	2 μL
RNA	X μL（≤1 μg）
nuclease-free H_2O	$23 - X$ μL

Incubate the samples at 70℃ for 10 min and then on ice for 10 min, then add the following components

5×RT buffer	8 μL
dNTP mixture（10 mmol/L）	4 μL
Ace	2 μL
RNase inhibitor （10 U/μL）	1 μL
total	40 μL

42℃ 1 h,94℃ 10 min,25℃ 2 min.

（4）Aliquot cDNA and frozen at −20℃.

2. Amplify V_H and V_L of anti-TNF − α：

（1）Design and synthesis of primers for V_H and V_L. Based on the characteristics of the Ig variable region gene sequence and the published mouse V_H and V_L gene sequences, design universal primers corresponding to different subclass Ig backbone sequences FR1 and FR4, respectively. The sequences are as follows：

V_H primers, 5′ sense（F1）: 5′− CAGTGGATAGACCGATGGGGG − 3′

V_H primers, 3′ reverse（R1）: 5′− ATGATGGTGTTAAGTCCTTCTGTA − 3′

V_L primers, 5′ sense（F2）: 5′− ATGGAGACAGACACACTCCTGCTAT − 3′

V_L primers, 3′ reverse（R2）: 5′− GGATACAGTTGGTGCAGCATCAGCCCGT − 3′

（2）Assemble one reaction containing the following reagents for each primer combination, using cDNA as template, and procedure is as follows：

10×PCR buffer	5 μL
2 mmol/L dNTPs	5 μL
25 mmol/L $MgSO_4$	3 μL
F1/F2	1 μL
R1/R2	1 μL
cDNA	1 μL（~200 ng）
KOD-Plus-Neo	1 μL
ddH_2O	33 μL
Total	50 μL

94℃ for 5 min, 30 cycles of 94℃ for 15 s, 56℃ for 15 s, 72℃ for 45 s, 72℃ for 10 min

（3）Run the products on a 2% agarose gel. Then cut out the 480 bp bands, and purify the DNA using *Recovery of DNA from Agarose Gels Kits*. Dissolve in 30 μL ddH_2O, then aliquot cDNA and frozen at −20℃.

(4) Sequencing the PCR product. Blast DNA sequence with Pubmed and IMGT; the sequences are correctly compared and then frozen at -20℃.

3. Overlap PCR to generate V_H - linker - V_L:

(1) Using overlapping PCR, the V_H and V_L are joined together by a linker. In order to facilitate the insertion of the expression vector, a restriction endonuclease is introduced at the $5'$ forward primer of V_H and the $3'$ reverse primer, respectively. The sequences are as follows:

V_H primers, $5'$ sense(F3): $5'-$ ATT<u>GCGGCCGC</u>TTATGGGGGTGTTGGGC $-3'$ (SalI)

V_H primers, $3'$ reverse (R3): $5'-$ <u>ACTACCGCCTCCACCACTACCGCCTCCACCAC TACCGCCTCCACC</u>GAGGTGCAGCTTCAGGAG $-3'$ (Gly4Ser)3

V_L primers, $5'$ sense(F4): $5'-$ <u>GGGTGGAGGCGGTAGTGGTGGAGGCGGTAGT GGTGGAGGCGGTAGT</u> CCGTTTGATCTCCAGCTT $-3'$ (Gly4Ser)3

V_L primers, $3'$ reverse (R4): $5'-$ ATT<u>GTCGAC</u>TCGAGTCACATTCTCAGCTC $-3'$ (NotI)

(2) Assemble one reaction containing the following reagents for each primer combination, and procedure is as follows:

10×PCR buffer	5 μL
2 mmol/L dNTPs	5 μL
25 mmol/L MgSO$_4$	3 μL
F3/F4	1 μL
R3/R4	1 μL
cDNA	1 μL(~200 ng)
KOD-Plus-Neo	1 μL
ddH$_2$O	33 μL
Total	50 μL

94℃ for 5 min, 30 cycles of 94℃ for 15 s, 56℃ for 15 s, 72℃ for 60 s, 72℃ for 10 min

(3) Run the products on a 2% agarose gel. Cut out the 550 bp bands, and purify the DNA and dissolve in 30 μL ddH$_2$O.

(4) Assemble one reaction containing the following reagents for F3 and R4 combination, using V_H-Linker and V_L-Linker as template, and procedure is as follows:

10×PCR buffer	5 μL
2 mmol/L dNTPs	5 μL
25 mmol/L MgSO$_4$	3 μL
F3	1 μL
R4	1 μL
cDNA	1 μL(~200 ng)
KOD-Plus-Neo	1 μL
ddH$_2$O	33 μL

| Total | 50 μL |

94℃ for 5 min, 30 cycles of 94℃ for 15 s, 56℃ for 15 s, 72℃ for 90 s, 72℃ for 10 min

(5) Run the products on a 1.5% agarose gel. Then cut out the 1,100 bp bands, and purify the DNA and dissolve in 30 μL ddH$_2$O.

4. Generate V$_H$ – linker – V$_L$ prokaryotic expression plasmid：

(1) Prepare the overlap scFv PCR products and the pGEX – 4T – 1 vector for cloning by performing restriction digests with *Sal*I and *Not*I, and procedure is as follows：

10×cut smart suffer	2 μL
*Sal*I	1 μL
*Not*I	1 μL
pGEX – 4T – 1/V$_H$ – linker – V$_L$	X μL (≤1 μg)
ddH$_2$O	20 – X μL
Total	20 μL

Incubate the samples at 37℃ for 2 h

(2) Run the products on a 1% agarose gel. Then cut out the 4,900 bp and 1,100 bp bands, and purify the DNA. Finally dissolve in 30 μL ddH$_2$O.

(3) T4 Generate pGEX – 4T – 1 – V$_H$ – linker – V$_L$ by T4 DNA ligase, and procedure is as follows：

10×T4 DNA ligase buffer	2 μL
pGEX – 4T – 1	1 μL
V$_H$ – linker – V$_L$	3 μL
T4 DNA Ligase	1 μL
ddH$_2$O	13 μL
total	20 μL

Incubate the samples at 16℃ for 16 h

(4) The ligation system is transformed into *E. coli* BL21 (DE3) strain. The ligated plasmids grow in agar plates containing ampicillin because of pGEX – 4T – 1 containing ampicillin resistance gene.

(5) Culture the positive clones, and the plasmid is extracted, and then identified by double digestion with *Sal*I and *Not*I. The positive clones show of 4,900 bp and 1,100 bp bands.

(6) Expand the success clones, and IPTG is added to LB when OD value is 0.6 – 0.8 to induce the expression of the target protein in bacteria. V$_H$ – linker – V$_L$(scFv) is purified by GST tag.

【Results】

1. scFv is successfully cloned from the hybridoma and inserted into the prokaryotic

expression vector pGEX − 4T − 1(Fig.28 − 1).

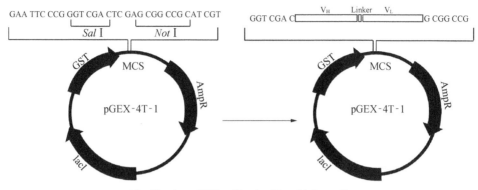

Fig.28 − 1   pGEX − 4T − 1 − V_H − Linker − V_L

2. The positive clone is identified by double digestion with *Sal*I and *Not*I. The positive clones show of 4,900 bp and 1,100 bp bands.

3. V_H − linker − V_L (scFv) is expressed successfully in bacteria.

【Precautions】

1. Primer design: design multiple sets of primers according to the immunoglobulin family so that the most monoclonal antibodies of V_H and V_L genes are amplified.

2. Two forms of scFv: the C terminal of V_H is connected to the N terminal of V_L, or the C terminal of V_L is connected to the N terminal of V_H.

3. Generation of plasmid: the product of overlapping PCR, V_H − Linker − V_L, is ligated to the T-vector, and then inserted into the expression vector.

【Questions】

1. What are the characteristics of the linker?

2. How to determine the quality of anti − TNF − α scFv?

3. Which expression vectors are inserted into the V_H − linker − V_L? What are the advantages and disadvantages of different expression vectors?

(Li Pingfei   Xi Xueyan)

第五篇
Chapter Five

常用的免疫相关疾病动物模型
Animal Models of Immuno-related Diseases

实验二十九　　豚鼠的过敏性休克反应模型

【原理】

豚鼠的速发型超敏反应属于Ⅰ型超敏反应,主要是由特异性 IgE 抗体介导,由肥大细胞和嗜碱性粒细胞释放大量过敏介质造成的一组症候群。当变应原(如马血清)首次进入机体后,可选择性地诱导特异性 B 细胞产生 IgE 抗体,IgE 以其 Fc 段与肥大细胞及嗜碱性粒细胞表面的高亲和性 IgE Fc 受体结合,从而使机体处于对该变应原致敏状态。当相同变应原再次进入机体时,通过与致敏肥大细胞和嗜碱性粒细胞表面的 IgE 抗体特异性结合,使膜表面 FcεRI 交联,触发致敏靶细胞脱颗粒,外排和分泌组胺、激肽等介质,数秒或数分钟内引起过敏性反应的症状(图 29-1)。

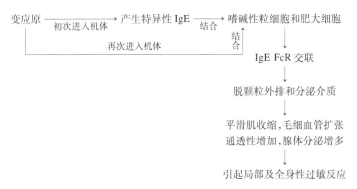

图 29-1　过敏性休克反应流程

【应用】

豚鼠是较好的动物过敏反应模型,因此可利用豚鼠来验证某种物质是否具有过敏原性质,也可筛选对抗Ⅰ型变态反应药物的模型,同时还可用来测定血清中 IgE 的效价。

【材料】

1. 豚鼠:体重 250 g 左右的成年雄性豚鼠,分成三组,每组 3 只

2. 过敏原的制备:

(1) 1∶5 和 1∶10 稀释马血清:取两支试管分别标号,用吸管吸取生理盐水,于第一管中加入 0.4 mL,第二支试管加入 0.25 mL;再用吸管吸取马血清,于第一管中加入 0.1 mL,混匀,则稀释度为 1∶5;用吸管吸取第一管中的稀释血清 0.25 mL 注入第二管,混匀,则稀释度为 1∶10。

(2) 1∶5 稀释鸡蛋清:取新鲜鸡蛋浸泡在 70%乙醇内,一天后用无菌注射器在无菌条件下经蛋壳吸取蛋清,再以无菌生理盐水以相同方法稀释至 1∶5。

3. 无菌生理盐水、无菌注射器、针头、3%品红溶液、小试管、吸管、试管架、记号笔、橡

皮乳头、酒精棉球等

【方法】

1. 用3%品红溶液将三组豚鼠分别编号,标记。

2. 豚鼠致敏注射(初次注射抗原):

(1) 豚鼠的抓取与固定:用左手手掌扣住豚鼠背部,抓住肩胛上方,拇指和食指扣住颈部,其余手指握持躯干,右手在下方将动物托起,手心向上,食指、中指、无名指夹住后腿,即可提取、固定。

(2) 豚鼠的皮下注射:用酒精棉球消毒豚鼠的下腹部,左手拇指和食指轻轻提起皮肤,右手持注射器于下腹部将针头刺入皮下,针头摆动无阻力,证明已进入皮下,推进药液。注入后,皮下呈扩散状隆起者为注射正确。

a. 第一组豚鼠皮下注射1:10稀释马血清0.2 mL。

b. 第二组豚鼠也皮下注射1:10稀释马血清0.2 mL。

c. 第三组豚鼠皮下注射生理盐水0.2 mL。

3. 豚鼠透发过敏注射(第二次注射抗原):

(1) 初次注射抗原2周后,给第一组豚鼠心内注射1:5稀释马血清1.5 mL。心内注射方法:一人抓取固定豚鼠,使其胸腹部朝上,另一人用左手触摸豚鼠左侧第4、5、6肋间,选择心跳最明显处将注射器刺入心脏(所用针头应细长,以免穿刺孔出血),出现回血后即将药物推入。

(2) 对照:

a 给第二组豚鼠心内注射1:5稀释鸡蛋清1.5 mL。

b 给第三组豚鼠心内注射1:5稀释马血清1.5 mL。

4. 注射后,在1~5 min内仔细观察豚鼠的症状(表29-1)。

表29-1　豚鼠过敏试验操作表

豚　　鼠	1	2	3
初次注射马血清(mL)	0.2	0.2	—
生理盐水(mL)	—	—	0.2
再次注射马血清(mL)	1.5	—	1.5
注射鸡蛋清(mL)	—	1.5	—

【结果】

数分钟内,第一组豚鼠出现兴奋不安、耸毛、抓鼻、打喷嚏、呃逆等症状,随后出现呼吸困难、痉挛性跳跃、抽搐、大小便失禁等症状,最后死亡。由于动物个体反应性不同,有的虽然出现上述症状但较轻,反应后可幸免死亡。而第二组和第三组豚鼠无任何过敏反应症状出现(图29-2)。

【注意事项】

1. 豚鼠选用敏感性较高的品系。

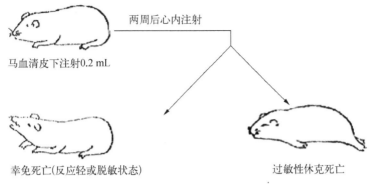

两周后心内注射

马血清皮下注射0.2 mL

幸免死亡(反应轻或脱敏状态)

过敏性休克死亡

图 29－2　豚鼠过敏反应示意图

2. 选择适宜浓度的变应原。

3. 实验过程中处理动物的手法应温和,以免动物受刺激过强产生激动而出现非特异性反应。

4. 不同个体动物的反应性有差异,每次不能只用一只动物,通常为了提高统计数据的精确性,每组使用 3 只动物。

5. 心内注射时,应在见到注射器内有回血后再注射抗原。

6. 再次注射变应原时,应做心内或静脉注射,使变应原直接进入血循环,才能引起明显的休克反应。

【思考题】

1. 速发型超敏反应的发生机制是什么?

2. 在第一组豚鼠中,若未发生过敏性休克,当再次心内注射同样的马血清时是否会发生过敏性休克?

3. 试述脱敏反应的原理。

（张秋萍）

Exp. 29　　Model of Anaphylaxis Shock in Guinea Pig

【Principle】

Hypersensitivity of immediate type in guinea pig is type I hypersensitivity, mediated by IgE antibody and release plenty allergic mediator by mast cells and basophils. When allergen (e. g. horse serum) is first injected into the body, it can induce specific B cells produce IgE antibody. IgE attaches to the high affinity IgE FcR on the surface of mast cells and basophils with its Fc, then makes the body sensitization to the allergen. When the same allergen is introduced to the body again, it attaches to the IgE which adheres on the surface of consequent cells, makes FcεRI cross-linking in the membrane surface, then guides the consequent cells degranulation and releases chemical substances, including histamine, kinin etc. These chemical substances can cause hypersensitivity symptoms within several seconds or minutes (Fig.29 − 1).

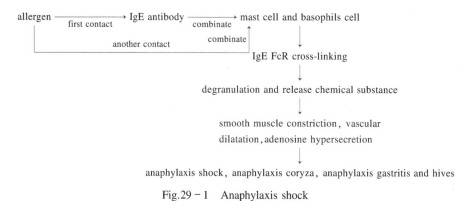

Fig.29 − 1　Anaphylaxis shock

【Application】

Guinea pig is a good model of animal hypersensitivity, so we can utilize it to analyze the anaphylactogen characteristic of some specific matter. We can also choose drugs which can count type I hypersensitivity. In addition, the titer of IgE in the serum can be determinated with this method.

【Materials】

1. Guinea pig: adult male guinea pigs (weight 250 g) are seperated into 3 groups, and 3 for each group

2. Allergen preparation:

(1) 1 : 5 and 1 : 10 diluted horse serum: mark 2 test tubes, drip physiological saline

0. 4 mL into first tube and 0. 25 mL into second tube with pipet. Then drip horse serum 0. 1 mL into first tube, jumble, the distant is 1 ：5; drip the diluted serum with first tube 0. 25 mL into the second tube, jumble, the dilution is 1 ：10.

(2) 1 ：5 diluted chicken egg albumin: drench fresh eggs into 70% alcohol. 24 hours later, get the egg albumin with aseptic syringe, dilute it to 1 ：5 with aseptic physiological saline by the same way.

3. Aseptic physiological saline, aseptic syringe, needle, 3% fuchsin solution, test tube, pipet, test tube rack, alcohol cotton ball, etc.

【Procedures】

1. Mark the 3 groups guinea pigs with 3% fuchsin solution.

2. Primary injection:

(1) Catch and immobization of guinea pig: catch the apostatize of guinea pig by left hand, thumb and forefinger clasp the neck, other fingers hold the body, right hand hold the bottom of animal, palm upwards.

(2) Guinea pigs' intradermally injection: pasteurize belly with alcohol cotton ball, thumb and forefinger carry the belly skin tightly, then inject the serum under the skin with syringe by the right hand.

a. The first group guinea pigs is injected 1 ：10 diluted horse serum 0. 2 mL.

b. The second group guinea pigs is injected 1 ：10 diluted horse serum 0. 2 mL.

c. The third group guinea pigs is injected saline 0. 2 mL.

3. Second injection:

(1) Two weeks later, the first group guinea pigs can be challenged by the intracardial injection with 1 ：5 diluted horse serum 1. 5 mL.

Method of intracardial injection: catch and immobility guinea pig, chest and belly upwards, touch the most obvious place with heart throb, thorn the syringe into the heart (the needle should tenuous and long to avoid bleed), inject the serum when the blood can be seen in the syringe.

(2) Controls:

a. The second group guinea pigs are given 1 ：5 diluted egg serum 1. 5 mL intracardiacally.

b. The third group guinea pigs are given 1 ：5 diluted horse serum 1. 5 mL intracardiacally.

4. Please observe the symptoms of the guinea pigs carefully within $1-5$ min(Tab. 29 − 1).

Tab. 29 − 1　Hypersensitivity of guinea pig

guinea	1	2	3
horse serum (mL)	0. 2	0. 2	—
N. S. (mL)	—	—	0. 2
horse serum again (mL)	1. 5	—	1. 5
egg albumin (mL)	—	1. 5	—

【Results】

Within few minutes, symptoms appear in the first group guinea, such as excitement, hair standing, scratching nose, sneezing, coughing, afterwards respiratory dyspnea, convulsive kick, defecation and then die. The second and third group guinea pigs have no hypersensitivity symptoms(Fig.29 - 2).

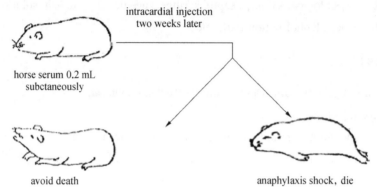

horse serum 0.2 mL
subctaneously

intracardial injection
two weeks later

avoid death

anaphylaxis shock, die

Fig.29 - 2   Hypersensitivity of guinea pig

【Precautions】

1. Select the high sensitive morality of guinea pigs.

2. Choose appropriate allergen.

3. The manipulation should be gently, otherwise animals would appear non-specific reaction.

4. 3 animals should be prepared for each group to obtain the statistical precision.

5. Serum should be injected after the blood can be seen in the syringe.

6. In the second injection, intracardial injection can cause obvious shock reaction.

【Questions】

1. What is the mechanism of immediate hypersensitivity?

2. In the first group guinea pigs, there is no anaphylaxis shock. If we inject to them the same horse serum, do you think that the anaphylaxis shock will appear?

3. What is the mechanism of anaphylaxis tolerance?

(Zhang Qiuping)

实验三十　　Ⅰ型超敏反应小鼠模型
——被动皮肤过敏反应

【原理】

过敏性疾病与超敏反应的发生密切相关,对人的生活造成很大的影响。它在人群中的发病率正逐年增加,这可能与现代社会生活条件和方式的改变,以及人们缺乏对有益微生物的接触有关。本实验介绍几种超敏反应的动物模型。

本实验将致敏小鼠的血清(内含丰富的 IgE 抗体)皮内注射于正常小鼠的腹壁或背部,每注射点形成一皮丘。IgE 与局部皮肤肥大细胞的 Fc 受体结合,使之被动致敏。

埃文斯蓝染料能结合在血液的白蛋白上。正常情况下,血管的内皮细胞连接紧密,白蛋白不会从血管渗出。当过敏发生时,内皮细胞间的紧密连接消失,白蛋白渗出到过敏局部。当过敏小鼠被注射埃文斯蓝染料时,染料同白蛋白一起渗出到过敏局部,形成蓝斑。

【应用】

判断皮肤过敏反应的程度,检验抗体或抗原的高敏感度。

【材料】

1. 天花粉
2. 4%氢氧化铝
3. 5%埃文斯蓝溶液(内含天花粉 1 mg)
4. 乙醚
5. 注射器、试管
6. 天平
7. 离心机
8. 剪刀
9. 刻度尺

【方法】

1. 抗血清制备:取健康小鼠 A,5 g 天花粉以 4% Al(OH)$_3$ 凝胶配成的混悬液,给小鼠 4 个足跖注射各 21 μL,共 84 μL。致敏后 10~14 天,处死动物后采得血液,经低速离心,分离血清,置冰箱 4℃备用。

2. 被动皮肤致敏及抗原攻击:另取健康小鼠 B,在乙醚麻醉下剪去背部的毛,将稀释的抗血清[稀释度可在(1∶20)~(1∶80)]皮内注射于鼠背部,至少注射两个稀释度,每一稀释度注射两点,每点 21 μL。48 h 后进行抗原攻击,静脉注射 115 μL 的 0.5%埃文斯蓝溶液(内含天花粉 1 mg)。20 min 后处死动物,翻转背部皮肤,测定蓝色反应斑的直径(图 30-1)。

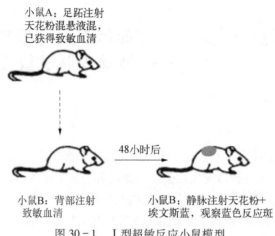

小鼠A：足跖注射
天花粉混悬液混，
已获得致敏血清

48小时后

小鼠B：背部注射
致敏血清

小鼠B：静脉注射天花粉+
埃文斯蓝，观察蓝色反应斑

图 30-1　Ⅰ型超敏反应小鼠模型

【结果观察】

蓝色反应斑的直径大小,判断皮肤过敏反应的程度。

【注意事项】

1. 本法是Ⅰ型超敏反应抗原常用的筛选方法,方法简便。

2. 注意假阳性的发生。有些药物可以增加血管通透性,也能得到阳性结果,应予排除。

3. 为使结果更加客观,可剪下蓝斑皮肤,每点以 5 mL 丙酮生理盐水溶液（3∶7, V/V）浸泡 48 h,离心,取上清,以 590 nm 测定光密度。

【思考题】

1. 抗原致敏的时间为什么选择在 10~14 天?

2. 为什么在抗原注射 20 min 以后进行抗原攻击检测?

（潘　勤）

Exp. 30　Murine Model of Type I Hypersensitivity Reaction — Passive Cutaneous Anaphylaxis Model

【Principle】

Allergic diseases, which are caused by hypersensitivity reaction, have great impact on the quality of people life. Cases are increasing in prevalence in humans, possibly due to the changed lifestyle conditions and the decreased exposure to beneficial microorganisms. Several animal models of hypersensitivity reaction are shown in this section.

Passive cutaneous anaphylaxis (PCA) is induced by intradermally injecting an exogenous IgE antibody specific against an antigen into abdominal wall or back of normal mice, forming a wheal at each injection point. IgE binds to the Fc receptor on mast cells. The Fc receptor signaling pathway in mast cells is activated leading to the overproduction of inflammatory mediators that trigger allergenic reactions and increased permeability of the local blood vessels.

Evans Blue is a dye that binds albumin. Under physiologic conditions the endothelium is impermeable to albumin, so Evans blue bound albumin remains restricted within blood vessels. In allergenic condition that promotes increased vascular permeability endothelial cells partially lose their close contacts and the endothelium becomes permeable to small proteins such as albumin. When the mice with allergy are intravenously injected with Evans blue, blueing of the skin at the site of the intradermal injection is evidence of the permeability reaction.

【Application】

Determine the degree of anaphylaxis reaction, IgE antibodies and allergens.

【Materials】

1. Trichosanthin
2. 4% aluminum hydroxide
3. 5% Evans blue solution (containing 1 mg of trichosanthin)
4. Ether
5. Syringe, test tube
6. Balance
7. Centrifuge
8. Scissors

9. Graduated ruler

【Procedures】

1. Antisera preparation: 5 g trichosanthin is mixed with 1 L of 4% Al(OH)$_3$ to form trichosanthin suspension. A mouse (Mouse A) is injected with trichosanthin suspension into four foot pads (21 μL per pad). 10－14 days after sensitization, the mouse is sacrificed and the blood is collected. The sera are separated after centrifugation and stored at 4℃.

2. Sensitization and antigen challenge: A mouse (Mouse B) is anesthetized with ether and cut off the back hair. The diluted antiserum [diluted at (1 : 20)－(1 : 80)] is intradermally injected into the mouse back. At least two dilutions of antiserum should be injected per mouse (21 μL/dilution/mouse). 48 hours after injection, antigen challenge is performed by intravenous administration with 115 μL of 0.5% Evans blue solution (containing 1 mg of trichosanthin). After 20 minutes, the mouse is sacrificed, and the diameter of blue reaction spot on the mouse skin is measured(Fig.30－1).

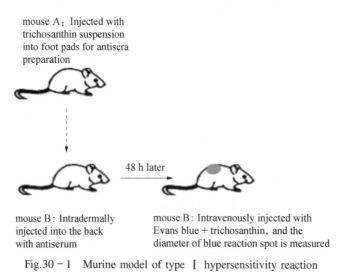

mouse A: Injected with trichosanthin suspension into foot pads for antisera preparation

48 h later

mouse B: Intradermally injected into the back with antiserum

mouse B: Intravenously injected with Evans blue + trichosanthin, and the diameter of blue reaction spot is measured

Fig.30－1   Murine model of type I hypersensitivity reaction

【Results】

Assessment of cutaneous anaphylaxis by determining the diameter of blue reaction spot on the mouse skin.

【Precautions】

1. PCA model is generally used for screening allergens causing anti-type I allergy. The method is simple.

2. Some drugs, which increase vascular permeability, may lead to false positive results in PCA model.

3. For additional assessment, the skin of the blue spot can be cut off, soaked in 5 mL of

acetone physiological saline solution ($3 : 7$, V/V) for 48 hours. After centrifugation, the supernatant is collected and the optical density at 590 nm is measured.

[Questions]

1. Why do we choose the time of antigen sensitization at $10 - 14$ days?
2. Why do we detect the antigen attack after 20min of antigen injection?

(Pan Qin)

实验三十一　Ⅱ型超敏反应豚鼠模型——Forssman 皮肤血管炎反应

【原理】

Ⅱ型超敏反应又名细胞毒性抗体反应，是由抗体与靶细胞表面抗原相结合而介导的。抗原可以是细胞膜自身成分，也可以是吸附在细胞表面的外源性抗原或半抗原，可通过活化补体系统或其他机制引起靶细胞损伤。

Forssman 抗原是存在于狗、马、猫、乌龟和绵羊等动物中的异嗜性抗原。绵羊红细胞（SRBC）免疫的兔可产生抗 SRBC 抗体（溶血素）。将这种抗体注射于豚鼠的皮内组织，在补体参与下引起红细胞的裂解，可引起皮肤血管炎，使血管通透性增加。皮肤血管炎反应轻重可以通过血管通透性来反映，亦称 Forssman 皮肤血管炎反应。

【应用】

建立Ⅱ型超敏反应模型，研究其病理过程。

【材料】

1. SRBC 保存液（Alsever's 液）：葡萄糖 2.05 g、氯化钠 0.42 g、柠檬酸钠 0.8 g、蒸馏水 100 mL，无菌过滤（G_5 漏斗）或 8 磅 10 min 灭菌后备用
2. SRBC：在无菌条件下自成年健康绵羊外颈静脉取血，室温下经 2 000 r/min 离心 10 min 得沉淀的细胞，用时用生理盐水洗涤，再按所需浓度稀释。稀释血细胞溶液可储存于 4℃
3. 生理盐水
4. 刻度尺
5. 剪刀
6. 注射器、试管
7. 离心机
8. 分光光度计

【方法】

1. 抗 SRBC 血清制备：将 10^9 个 SRBC 混悬于 1 mL 磷酸盐缓冲液中。给正常兔静脉注射 SRBC（$5×10^8$ SRBC/kg），隔天 1 次，共 10 次。于最后一次注射 14 天后收集兔血清，即抗 SRBC 血清，亦即溶血素。
2. 抗血清接种及超敏反应的观察：取健康豚鼠，剪去背部的毛，将 1∶8 生理盐水稀释的抗血清皮内注射于背部，每点 0.1 mL。可根据实验要求，注射多个稀释度的抗血清，每个稀释度至少注射两点。24 h 后可见注射局部有炎症反应。静脉注射 0.5% 埃文斯蓝

染料1 mL,30 min后,注射局部有一明显的蓝斑。处死动物,用刻度尺测定皮肤蓝斑的直径(图31-1)。

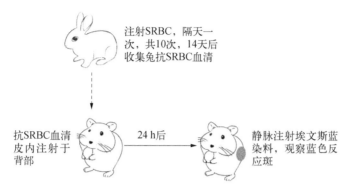

图31-1　Ⅱ型超敏反应豚鼠模型

【结果】

根据皮肤蓝斑的直径,判断血管炎症程度。

【注意事项】

为使结果更加客观,可剪下蓝斑皮肤,每点以5 mL丙酮生理盐水溶液(3∶7,V/V)浸泡48 h,离心,取上清,以590 nm测定光密度。

【思考题】

本实验的影响因素有哪些?

（潘　勤）

Exp. 31   Guinea Pig Type Ⅱ Hypersensitivity Reaction — Forssman Cutaneous Vasculitis Response

【Principle】

Type II hypersensitivity reaction, also known as cytotoxic hypersensitivity, is mediated by the binding of antibodies to antigens on the surface of target cells. The antigen may be a component of the cell membrane, an exogenous antigen or hapten adsorbed on the cell surface. When antibody binds to the antigen on cell surface, the binding causes damage to the target cell by activating the complement system or other mechanisms.

The Forssman antigen is a glycolipid heterophil protein and a type of heterogenetic antigen found in certain animals like dogs, horses, cats, turtles and sheep. Rabbit immunized with sheep red blood cells (SRBC) produces anti-SRBC antibodies (hemolysin). Intradermally injecting anti-SRBC antibodies into a guinea pig leads to lysis of red blood cells, increased vascular permeability and vasculitis of the skin in site of injection, also known as Forssman cutaneous vasculitis response.

【Application】

To study and assess the pathological process of type II hypersensitivity reaction.

【Materials】

1. SRBC preservation solution (Alsever's solution): glucose 2.05 g, NaCl 0.42 g, sodium citrate 0.8 g, distilled water 100 mL, then aseptically filtered (G_5 funnel) or autoclaved (8 lbs for 10 minutes)

2. SRBC: Under aseptic conditions, blood is taken from the external jugular vein of an adult sheep. The blood is centrifuged (2,000 r/min, 10 min) at room temperature. Saline is used to wash and resuspend the blood cells. The SRBC is stored at 4℃

3. Saline

4. Scissors

5. Syringe, test tube

6. Centrifuge

7. Graduated ruler

8. Spectrophotometer

【Procedures】

1. Anti-SRBC sera preparation: 10^9 SRBCs are suspended in 1 mL of phosphate buffer.

Rabbits are injected (5×10^8 SRBC/kg) intravenously once every other day for 10 times. Rabbit serum is collected 14 days after the last injection. The serum is anti-SRBC serum, also known as hemolysin.

2. Antisera inoculation and observation of type Ⅱ hypersensitivity reaction: A guinea pig is cut off the hair on the back, and intradermally injected with the antiserum (anti-serum: saline $V/V = 1 : 8$, 0. 1 mL/injection point). Multiple dilutions of antiserum can be injected according to the experimental requirements. Each dilution is performed in duplicate. After 24 hours of injection, a local inflammatory reaction in the site of injection occurs. Half an hour after intravenous injection with 1 mL of 0. 5% Evans blue solution, there are apparent blue spots in the injection site. The diameter of the skin blue spots is measured by a graduated ruler(Fig.31 - 1).

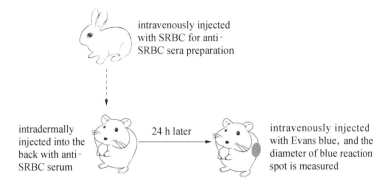

Fig.31 - 1   Guinea pig model of type Ⅱ hypersensitivity reaction

【Results】

According to the diameter of the skin blue spot, the severity of vascular inflammation is assessed.

【Precautions】

For additional assessment, the skin of the blue spot can be cut off, soaked in 5 mL of acetone physiological saline solution (3 : 7, V/V) for 48 hours. After centrifugation, the supernatant is collected and the optical density at 590 nm is measured.

【Question】

What are the factors influencing the experimental results?

(Pan Qin)

实验三十二　Ⅲ型超敏反应动物模型——Arthus 反应

【原理】

Ⅲ型超敏反应又称免疫复合物型变态反应,是指抗原抗体复合物沉积于组织中而引起的细胞组织损伤。

Ⅲ型超敏反应动物模型需要有抗原的持续存在。将抗原物质反复注射动物,抗原与相应抗体结合形成游离的免疫复合物,在一定条件下这种复合物沉积在血管壁基膜或组织间隙,通过激活补体、中性粒细胞或血小板,造成沉积部位炎症变化。这一反应亦称 Arthus 反应。

【应用】

建立Ⅲ型超敏反应动物模型,研究Ⅲ型超敏反应病理过程。

【材料】

1. 卵白蛋白
2. Freund's 完全佐剂
3. 1 mL 注射器
4. 刻度尺

【方法】

1. 将经 3 次重结晶的卵白蛋白乳化于 Freund's 完全佐剂中,乳化必须充分。
2. 给兔每周肌肉注射 1 mL 卵白蛋白乳剂,共 4 次。
3. 最后 1 次注射后的第 9 天,背部剪毛;第 10 天背部皮内注射 10% 卵白蛋白,每点注射量为 0.2 mL。
4. 抗原攻击后 2 h、3 h、4 h、6 h、8 h、12 h、24 h 观察每个注射点局部皮肤红肿的最大直径与反应的程度,求其平均值。

反应程度标准分级:

+++:2 h 或 5 h 明显充血、出血,呈融合状;24 h 明显出血性变色。

++:2 h 或 5 h 中度充血、出血,呈斑块状;24 h 中度出血性变色。

+:2 h 或 5 h 轻度充血、出血;24 h 轻度出血性变色。

−:2 h 或 24 h 均无反应。

【结果】

根据兔背部皮肤的充血、出血等病变分析 Arthus 反应的严重程度。

【注意事项】

1. 卵白蛋白并与 Freund's 完全佐剂应乳化充分。

2. 可以大鼠代替兔。大鼠 Arthus 反应形成所需肌肉注射卵白蛋白的次数比兔多,每鼠每周肌肉注射 0.5 mL,共 6 次,前 3 次为卵白蛋白-Freund's 完全佐剂,后 3 次卵白蛋白-Freund's 不完全佐剂。但大鼠 Arthus 反应不如兔严重。

【思考题】

1. 本实验除了卵白蛋白,还可以用什么物质进行 Arthus 反应的检测?

2. 试举例说明人类常见的 Ⅳ 型超敏反应疾病及其原理。

（潘 勤）

Exp. 32   Rabbit Type Ⅲ Hypersensitivity Reaction — Arthus Reaction

【Principle】

Type Ⅲ hypersensitivity reaction, also known as immune complex type of allergy, refers to cell tissue damage caused by deposition of antigen-antibody complexes in tissues.

The formation of this model requires the persistence of antigens in an animal by repetitive injection with antigens. The antigens combine with the corresponding antibodies to form immune complexes. The immune complexes are deposited in the basement membrane or tissue space of the vascular wall, and cause inflammation by activating complement, neutrophils or platelets at the deposition site. This reaction is also known as the Arthus reaction.

【Application】

To study and assess the pathological process of type Ⅲ hypersensitivity reaction.

【Materials】

1. Ovalbumin
2. Freund's complete adjuvant
3. 1 mL syringe
4. Graduated ruler

【Procedures】

1. The ovalbumin, which is recrystallized 3 times, emulsified sufficiently in Freund's complete adjuvant.

2. A rabbit is intramuscularly injected with 1 mL of ovalbumin emulsion per week for total 4 times.

3. On the 9th day after the last injection, the back hair of the rabbit is cut off. On the 10th day, 10% ovalbumin is intradermally injected into the rabbit back (0.2 mL/injection point).

4. The maximum diameter and reaction degree of local skin redness at each point are observed at 2 h, 3 h, 4 h, 6 h, 8 h, 12 h and 24 h after antigen challenge, and the average value is evaluated.

Standard grade of reaction:

+++: Obvious hyperemia, hemorrhage, fusion after 2 h or 5 h; 24 h of obvious hemorrhagic discoloration.

++: Moderate hyperemia, hemorrhage, plaque after 2 h or 5 h; 24 h of moderate hemorrhagic discoloration.

+: Mild hyperemia, hemorrhage after 2 h or 5 h; 24 h of mild hemorrhagic discoloration.

-: No reaction at 2 h or 24 h.

【Results】

According to the degree of hyperemia and hemorrhage on the skin, the severity of Arthus reaction is assessed.

【Precautions】

1. Sufficient emulsification of ovalbumin in Freund's complete adjuvant is required for Arthus reaction.

2. A rat can also be used in this experiment. The amount of ovalbumin used for a rat is more than that for a rabbit. A rat is intramuscularly injected with 0.5 mL per week for 6 times. The mixtures of ovalbumin-Freund's complete adjuvant are used for first 3 injections, and the mixtures of ovalbumin-Freund's incomplete adjuvant are used for last 3 injections. However, the rat Arthus response is not as severe as that in rabbit.

【Questions】

1. Besides ovalbumin, what other substances can be used in this experiment for the detection of Arthus reaction?

2. Give examples of human common type IV hypersensitive diseases and their mechanisms.

(Pan Qin)

实验三十三　Ⅳ型超敏反应小鼠模型——二硝基氟苯诱导的迟发型变态反应

【原理】

Ⅳ型超敏反应亦称迟发型变态反应（DTH），其发生与抗体和补体无关，主要由 T 细胞介导的免疫损伤所致。其病理学表现为单个核细胞浸润、细胞变性和坏死为特征的局部超敏反应性炎症。该反应进程较迟缓，一般于再次接触抗原后 48~72 h 发生，故称为迟发型变态反应。其反应迟缓的原因是体内致敏 T 细胞再次与相应抗原接触而被激活并产生淋巴因子，以及足够多的单个核细胞汇聚炎症区域，这些均需一定时间。

二硝基氟苯（DNFB）是一种半抗原，将其溶液涂抹于小鼠腹壁皮肤后，DNFB 与皮肤蛋白质结合成完全抗原，由此刺激 T 淋巴细胞增殖成致敏淋巴细胞。4~7 天后将其再次涂抹于小鼠皮肤，可使局部产生迟发型变态反应（水肿）。

【应用】

建立Ⅳ型超敏反应动物模型，研究Ⅳ型超敏反应病理过程。检测免疫缺陷或使用免疫抑制剂的人能否对新引入的抗原发生细胞免疫反应。

【材料】

1. 丙酮麻油溶液：丙酮与麻油以 1：1 体积混匀
2. 1% DNFB 溶液：DNFB 50 mg 溶于 5 mL 丙酮—麻油溶液
3. 天平
4. 剪刀
5. 卡尺（0.01~12.5 mm）
6. 8 mm 皮革打孔器

【方法】

1. 致敏：小鼠腹部去毛，约 3 cm×3 cm。将 1% DNFB 溶液均匀涂抹在小鼠腹部，必要时次日再强化 1 次。
2. 迟发型变态反应：致敏后第 5 天，将 1% DNFB 溶液 10 μL 均匀涂抹于小鼠右耳（两面）进行抗原攻击。攻击后 24 h，用卡尺测量两只耳朵的耳郭厚度，颈椎脱白处死小鼠，剪下左右耳郭，用打孔器取下直径 8 mm 的耳片称重。

【结果】

1. 估算左右耳郭厚度改变（ΔT）：

$$\Delta T = 右耳耳郭厚度 - 左耳耳郭厚度$$

2. 估算左右耳片肿胀度(ΔW)：

$$\Delta W = 右耳片重量 - 左耳片重量$$

【注意事项】

1. 其他抗原也可成功地用于 DTH 反应动物模型，包括卵清蛋白、卡介苗（BCG）、各种半抗原和微生物成分。

2. 该模型的优势之一是可通过同一只小鼠的两只耳朵进行比对，评估 DTH 反应的程度。

3. 8 mm 耳片也可以保存在干冰或液氮上，以进行蛋白质或 RNA 提取。

【思考题】

为什么 DNFB 能引起Ⅳ型超敏反应？

（潘　勤）

Exp. 33 Mouse Type Ⅳ Hypersensitivity Reaction — Dinitrofluorobenzene-induced Delayed Type Hypersensitivity

【Principle】

Type Ⅳ hypersensitivity reaction, also known as delayed type hypersensitivity (DTH), occurs independently of antibodies or complements, and is mainly caused by T cell-mediated immune damage. Type Ⅳ hypersensitivity is characterized by local inflammation including mononuclear cell infiltration and cell degeneration and necrosis. The progress of the reaction is slow, and generally occurs in 48 – 72 h after reexposure to the antigen. The reason for its slow response is that it takes a certain time for the sensitized T cells to respond to the antigen and to produce lymphokines, leading to aggregation of mononuclear cells within the inflammatory sites.

Dinitrofluorobenzene (DNFB) is a kind of hapten. When the DNFB solution is applied to the abdominal skin of a mouse, DNFB binds to the skin protein and forms a complete antigen, thereby sensitizing T cells. 4 – 7 days later, DNFB is applied to the mouse skin again. It causes DTH reaction (edema).

【Application】

To study and assess the pathological process of type Ⅳ hypersensitivity reaction. To detect whether a person with immunodeficiency or subjected to immunosuppressive agent treatment has a cellular immune response to a newly introduced antigen.

【Materials】

    1. Acetone and sesame oil solution: acetone mixed with sesame oil (1 : 1, *V/V*)

    2. 1% DNFB solution: DNFB 50 mg mixed with 5 mL of acetone sesame oil solution

    3. Balance

    4. Scissors

    5. Calipers (dial thickness gauge 0. 01 – 12. 5 mm)

    6. 8 mm leather hole punch

【Procedures】

    1. Sensitization: a mouse is cut off the hair on abdomen, and about 3 cm×3 cm size of hair is removed. 1% DNFB solution is applied to the mouse abdomen. If necessary, 1% DNFB can be applied again to the abdomen the next day for strengthening antigen

sensitization.

2. DTH reaction: 5 days after sensitization, 10 μl of 1% DNFB solution is applied to the right ear (both sides) of the mouse for challenge. 24 h after the challenge, measure pinna thickness for both ears using calipers. The mouse is sacrificed. Remove the left and right pinnas. Place each individual pinna on a cork board and use the 8 mm leather punch to remove the central portion of the pinna. Weigh each 8 mm pinna punch using an analytical scale.

【Results】

1. Calculate the change in pinna thickness (ΔT) using the following equation:

ΔT = (pinna thickness of the right ear) − (pinna thickness of the left ear)

2. Calculate the change in pinna weight (ΔW):

ΔW = (pinna weight of the right ear) − (pinna weight of the left ear)

【Precautions】

1. Other common antigens have also been successfully used for the DTH reaction, including ovalbumin, bacille Calmette-Guérin (BCG), various haptens and microbial constituents.

2. One of the advantages of this model is the ability to evaluate the DTH reaction using experimental and control ears from the same animal.

3. The 8 mm pinna punches can also be frozen on dry ice or by liquid nitrogen and manually homogenized for protein or RNA extraction.

【Question】

Why does DNFB cause Type Ⅳ hypersensitivity reaction?

(Pan Qin)

实验三十四　小鼠实验性自身免疫性脑脊髓炎的诱导

【原理】

正常情况下,中枢神经系统是一个免疫豁免区,外周的免疫细胞并不会通过血脑屏障进入中枢神经系统发挥其免疫作用。但在疾病情况下,脊髓髓鞘蛋白通过受损的血脑屏障进入到外周免疫器官,诱导免疫应答,然后特异性致敏的 CD4$^+$T 细胞由外周进入中枢神经系统,导致中枢神经系统内出现大量免疫细胞浸润以及脊髓脱髓鞘的病理表现。在诱导小鼠实验性自身免疫性脑脊髓炎(EAE)模型过程中,首先对小鼠进行皮下抗原免疫,同时破坏血脑屏障的通透性,当外周特异性致敏的淋巴细胞通过受损的血脑屏障进入中枢神经系统,对神经元和髓鞘造成损伤,产生相应的疾病症状(图 34-1)。

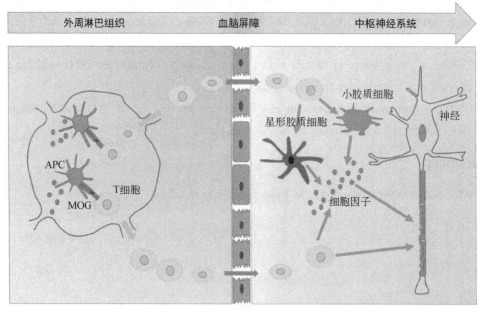

图 34-1　小鼠 EAE 模型发病示意图

APC:抗原提呈细胞;MOG:髓鞘少突胶质细胞糖蛋白

【应用】

EAE 模型是一个理想的人类多发性硬化(MS)的动物模型,可用于研究人类 MS 的发生、发展等一系列科学问题。

【材料】

1. SPF 级 6~8 周龄雌性 C57 小鼠
2. 免疫抗原：MOG_{35-55}
3. 免疫佐剂：完全弗氏佐剂（CFA），结核分枝杆菌 MTB
4. 百日咳毒素（PTX）
5. 无菌 PBS
6. 麻药：0.5% 戊巴比妥钠
7. 无菌玻璃注射器
8. 一次性无菌三通管
9. 1 mL 一次性无菌注射器

【方法】

1. 注射 PTX：小鼠于免疫前 30 min 腹腔注射 PTX（用 PBS 稀释至 1 ng/μL），200 μL/只。

2. 麻醉小鼠：腹腔注射 0.5% 戊巴比妥钠进行麻醉，300 μL/只。

3. 抗原免疫：待小鼠完全麻醉后，皮下注射抗原进行免疫。注射点为小鼠背部中线两侧近腋窝淋巴结和腹股沟淋巴结皮下的 4 个点（图 34-2），每点注射 50 μL，共 200 μL/只。

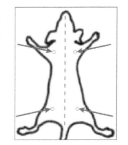

图 34-2　皮下免疫位点示意图

免疫抗原的制备：

（1）A 液：将 MOG_{35-55} 溶于无菌 PBS 中，至浓度为 2 mg/mL。

（2）B 液：将 MTB 溶于 CFA 中，至浓度为 5 mg/mL。

（3）将 A 液与 B 液按 1:1 混合，然后吸入一无菌玻璃注射器，然后依次接上三通管和另一注射器，旋紧每个接口。

（4）乳化：冰上来回抽吸注射器 45 min（15 min×3），使混合液充分乳化，乳化完全的乳液滴入水中不扩散。

4. 注射 PTX：造模 48 h 后，重复腹腔注射 PTX 一次，剂量同步骤 1。

【结果】

EAE 发病严重程度的评价：造模后每天对小鼠发病情况和临床症状进行评分和记录：0 分，无临床症状；0.5 分，尾巴部分无力或尾端下垂；1 分，尾巴完全瘫痪；2 分，运动失调，后肢轻度瘫痪；2.5 分，单后肢瘫痪；3 分，双后肢瘫痪；3.5 分，双后肢瘫痪，前肢无力；4 分，前肢瘫痪；5 分，垂死。

【注意事项】

1. 雌性小鼠对 EAE 模型的诱导更为敏感。
2. 抗原乳化要充分。
3. 抗原的免疫部位尽可能靠近淋巴结。

【思考题】

1. 有哪些原因可能影响小鼠发病的严重程度?
2. 本实验中,为什么要先进行百日咳毒素的注射?

（曾凡帆　郑　芳）

Exp. 34   Induction of Mouse Experimental Autoimmune Encephalomyelitis

【Principle】

Under normal circumstances, the central nervous system is an immune exemption zone, that means peripheral immune cells could not enter the central nervous system through the blood-brain barrier to exert their immune function. However, in the case of disease, the spinal myelin protein somehow enters the peripheral immune organs through the damaged blood-brain barrier, and then the specifically sensitized CD4$^+$ T cells enter the central nervous system from the periphery to exert immune response, resulting in large immune cell infiltration and demyelination. In the process of inducing mouse experimental autoimmune encephalomyelitis (EAE) model, we subcutaneously immunize the mouse with specific antigen, and simultaneously destroy the permeability of the blood-brain barrier. Then the specific sensitized lymphocytes from periphery enter the central nervous system through the damaged blood-brain barrier to exert a specific immune response, and eventually the EAE symptoms appears (Fig.34 − 1).

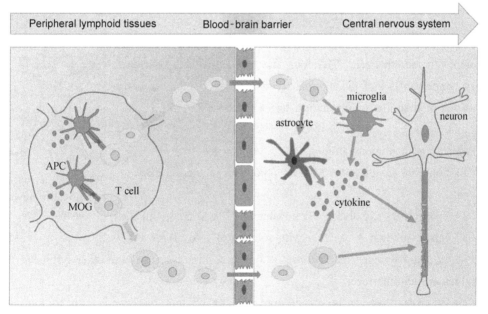

Fig.34 − 1   Pathogenesis of mouse EAE

APC: antigen presenting cell; MOG: myelin oligodendrocyte glycoprotein

【Application】

The EAE model is an ideal animal model of human multiple sclerosis (MS), which can be used to study a series of scientific problems such as the occurrence and development of human MS.

【Materials】

1. 6 – 8 weeks old female SPF（specific pathogen free）C57BL/6 mice

2. Immune antigen：MOG$_{35-55}$

3. Immune adjuvant：complete freund's adjuvant（CFA）, mycobacterium tuberculosis（MTB）

4. Pertussis toxin（PTX）

5. Sterile PBS

6. Anesthesia：0.5% pentobarbital sodium

7. Sterile glass syringes

8. Sterile three-limb tubes

9. 1 mL of disposable sterile syringes

【Procedures】

1. Injection of PTX：intraperitoneal injection of 200 μL PTX（diluted with PBS to 1 ng/μL）half an hour before immunization.

2. Anesthesia：intraperitoneal injection of 0.5% pentobarbital sodium, 300 μL per mouse.

3. Immunization：Subcutaneous immunization when the mice are completely anesthetized. The four injection points are near the axillary lymph nodes and the inguinal lymph nodes, which on both sides of the median line of the mouse back（Fig.34 – 2）, 50 μL for each point.

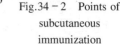

Fig.34 – 2 Points of subcutaneous immunization

Preparation of immune antigen：

（1）Solution A：dissolve MOG$_{35-55}$ powder in sterile PBS to 2 mg/mL.

（2）Solution B：dissolve MTB powder in CFA to 5 mg/mL

（3）Inhale solution A together with solution B（A : B = 1 : 1）into a sterile glass syringe, then connect it to a three-limb tubes and the other syringe in turn, and tightened each interface.

（4）Emulsify：syringe is sucked into ice for 45 min back and forth to thoroughly emulsification of the mixed liquid. Ways to test emulsification done：the emulsion drops on the water but indiffusion.

4. Injection of PTX：repeat intraperitoneal injection of PTX 48 h after immunization with the same dose as in procedure 1.

【Results】

Evaluation of EAE disease severity

Scoring and recording the incidence and clinical symptoms of every mouse the day after induction: 0 points, no clinical signs; 0.5 points, partially limp tail; 1 points, paralyzed tail; 2 points, loss in coordinated movement, hind limb paresis; 2.5 points, one hind limb paralyzed; 3 points, both hind limbs paralyzed; 3.5 points, hind limbs paralyzed, weakness in forelimbs; 4 points, forelimbs paralyzed; 5 points, moribund.

【Precautions】

1. The female mice are more sensitive to the induction of the EAE model than the male mice.

2. Antigen emulsification.

3. The immunization points, it is better to inject close to lymph nodes.

【Questions】

1. What factors may affect the severity of the disease in mouse?

2. In this experiment, why should the injection of PTX be carried out first?

(Zeng Fanfan　Zheng Fang)

Chapter Six

免疫学标记技术
Immunolabeling Technique

实验三十五　　酶联免疫吸附试验

【原理】

酶联免疫吸附试验(ELISA)的基本原理是：① 使抗原或抗体结合到某种固相载体表面,并保持其免疫活性。② 使抗原或抗体与某种酶连接成酶标抗原或抗体,这种酶标抗原或抗体既保留其免疫活性,又保留酶的活性。在测定时,把受检标本(测定其中的抗体或抗原)和酶标抗原或抗体按不同的步骤与固相载体表面的抗原或抗体起反应。用洗涤的方法洗去未结合的组分,最后结合在固相载体上的酶量与标本中受检物质的量成一定的比例。加入酶反应的底物后,底物被酶催化变为有色产物,产物的量与标本中受检物质的量直接相关,故可根据颜色反应的深浅进行定性或定量分析。由于酶的催化频率很高,故可极大地放大反应效果,从而使测定方法达到很高的敏感度。此法的特异性及灵敏度与荧光及同位素标记相似,但其方法较以上两者简便,且不需特殊贵重仪器。因此,这项技术目前正越来越广泛地被应用到医学等各个领域中。

ELISA 有许多种不同的方法,常用的基本方法有：直接法、间接法、双抗体夹心法和抗原竞争法。图 35-1 为 ELISA 间接法。

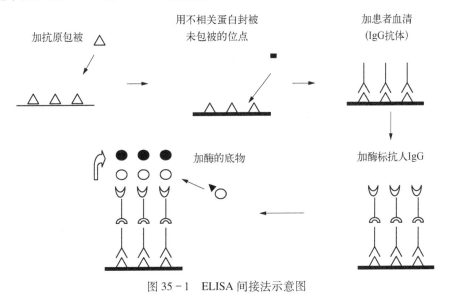

图 35-1　ELISA 间接法示意图

【应用】

ELISA 是一非常敏感的实验方法,可用于检测抗原或抗体,协助疾病的诊断。当与标准曲线联用时,还可定量检测样品中的抗原或抗体的含量,如 ELISA 常用于检测乙肝患者血清中 HBsAb。

以下以检测活动性结核患者血清中抗结核杆菌 IgG 抗体为例介绍 ELISA 间接法。

【材料】

1. 抗原：PPD(纯蛋白衍生物，结核杆菌培养物滤液中纯化的部分结核杆菌蛋白)
2. 15% 牛血清
3. 待测患者血清、结核患者阳性血清及阴性对照血清
4. 辣根过氧化物酶标记羊抗人 IgG 抗体
5. 0.05 mol/L pH 9.6 碳酸盐缓冲液；pH 7.4 吐温—磷酸盐缓冲液；pH 5.0 磷酸盐—柠檬酸缓冲液；邻苯二胺、30%过氧化氢、2 mol/L 硫酸
6. 聚苯乙烯微量塑料板，酶标测定仪等

【方法】

1. 包被抗原：抗原用 0.05 mol/L pH9.6 碳酸盐缓冲液以最适浓度(20 μg/mL)稀释后，加入聚苯乙烯微量塑料板孔中，每孔 100 μL，置 4℃过夜。倒空包被液后用 pH 7.4 吐温—磷酸盐缓冲液洗 3 次，每次 3 min。

2. 封闭：每孔加 100 μL 15%牛血清，于 37℃ 2 h。同法洗 3 次。

3. 加待检血清：用 pH 7.4 吐温—磷酸盐缓冲液以 1∶100 稀释，每孔加入 100 μL。每份标本加 2 孔，每板设阳性及阴性对照血清，阳性及阴性对照血清均按 1∶100 稀释。置 37℃ 40 min 后，倒空液体，用 pH 7.4 吐温—磷酸盐缓冲液洗 3 次，每次 3 min。

4. 加酶(如辣根过氧化物酶)联羊抗人 IgG：每孔加入适当工作浓度的酶联羊抗人 IgG 100 μL，置 37℃ 30 min。倒空液体后如上洗 3 次。

5. 加底物：每孔加入新鲜配制的底物(如辣根过氧化物酶的底物：100 mL pH5.0 磷酸盐—柠檬酸缓冲液加邻苯二胺 40 mg，30% H_2O_2 0.2 mL) 溶液 100 μL，放 37℃数分钟显色，适时观察颜色的变化，最后每孔加一滴 2 mol/L H_2SO_4 终止反应，肉眼观察或用酶标测定仪测定各孔光密度。

【结果】

肉眼观察，阴性血清无色或微黄色。阳性血清明显黄色。待测标本明显高于阴性而呈黄色则可判断阳性。如测定光密度，待测样品光密度(OD_{490})为阴性血清光密度值的 2 倍以上可判为阳性。

【注意事项】

1. 包被液通常用新鲜配制的 pH 9.6 碳酸盐缓冲液，包被板一经洗涤，则不宜存放过长时间。
2. 包被和温育均应将固相载体放至湿盒内进行。

【思考题】

为什么标记一种抗抗体可以检测多对抗原抗体系统？

(章晓联)

Exp. 35　Enzyme-Linked Immunosorbent Assay （ELISA）

〔Principle〕

The basic principle of ELISA is as follows: ① make antigen or antibody binding to a solid phase carrier surface, and maintain its immune activity. ② make antigen or antibody and an enzyme into a binding enzyme labelled antigen or antibody, this enzyme labelled antigen or antibody both retain its immune activity, and retain the activity of the enzyme. In assay, the tested specimen (antibody or antigen) and the enzyme-labeled antigen or antibody react with the antigen or antibody on the surface of the solid phase carrier in different steps. The unbound components is washed by washing method, and the amount of enzyme bound on the solid phase carrier is proportional to the amount of material tested in the specimen. After adding the substrate of the enzyme reaction, the substrate is catalyzed by the enzyme into colored products. The amount of the product is directly related to the amount of the substance tested in the specimen, so qualitative or quantitative analysis can be conducted according to the depth of the color reaction. Because the catalytic frequency of enzyme is very high, the reaction effect can be greatly amplified, so that the determination method achieves a high sensitivity. The specificity and sensitivity of this method are similar to those of fluorescence and isotope labelling method, however this method is simpler and does not require special expensive instrument. ELISA is now widely used in many areas in the medicine.

There are many different approaches to ELISAs. They are typically performed as a direct or an indirect method (Fig. 35 − 1), but can also be performed as a double antibodies

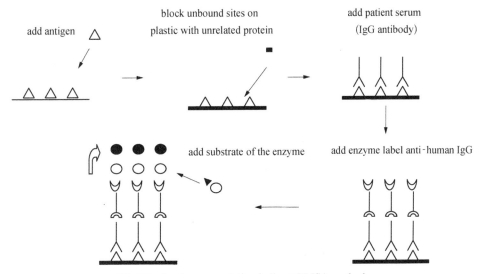

Fig.35 − 1　A representative indirect ELISA method

sandwich method and a competition assay. Here we introduce an indirect ELISA method.

【Application】

ELISA is a very sensitive laboratory method and can be quantitative when used in conjunction with standard curves. It can quantify the amount of antigen or antibody present in a given sample. Below is the example of the indirect ELISA. For example, ELISA is usually used for detect serum HBsAb. This experiment is to determine the anti-TB IgG whether present in the diagnostic patient serum.

【Materials】

1. Antigen: PPD (purified protein derivative, which is a tuberculoprotein derived by fraction of a broth culture filtrate of *Mycobacterium tuberculosis*)

2. 15% calf serum

3. Diagnostic patient serum (unknown Ab); tuberculosis (TB) patients positive serum and negative control serum

4. Horseradish peroxidase (HRP) labelled sheep anti-human IgG

5. 0.05 mol/L, pH 7.4 tween-phosphate buffered saline (PBS); pH 9.6 carbonate buffer; pH 5.0 citrate-phosphate buffer saline (PBS); o(orth)-diaminobenzene (OPD), 30% hydroperoxide (H_2O_2), 2 mol/L sulfate acid

6. Microtiter plate; plate reader, etc.

【Procedures】

1. Coat the wells of the microtiter plate with antigen: 100 μL 0.05 mol/L carbonate buffer diluted antigen (pH 9.6) is added into each well, incubated at 4℃ for overnight. Then empty the wells and wash the wells with tween-phosphate-buffered saline (pH 7.4) for three times, each time for 3 min.

2. Block each well with 100 μL 15% calf serum at 37℃ for 2 h. Wash 3 times.

3. Add patient serum (unknown Ab), TB patient's positive serum and negative control serum, 100 μL/well, each antibody is diluted as 1 : 100 with pH 7.4 tween-phosphate-buffer saline. Each sample well is duplicate. Incubate the microtiter plate at 37℃ for 40 min. Then empty the wells and wash with pH 7.4 tween-phosphate-buffered saline for three times, each time for 5 min.

4. 100 μL diluted enzyme (e.g. HRP)-labelled anti-human IgG is added into each well and incubated at 37℃ for 30 min. And then empty the wells and wash as before.

5. Add the substrate of the enzyme [freshly prepared substrate: 100 mL pH 5.0 citrate-phosphate-buffered saline plus 40 mg, o(orth)-diaminobenzene (OPD), 0.2 mL 30% H_2O_2], incubate at 37℃ for several minutes until color is appeared. Add 2 mol/L sulfate acid to end the reaction. Measure the color change by the plate reader.

[Results]

Observe the color changes. Yellow color represents "+" result, while the weak or white color represents "-" result. Usually if the absorbance value of the sample at OD_{490} is more than twice as that of the negative control sample, it can be represented as "+" result.

[Precautions]

1. The carbonate buffers (pH 9.6) are usually used as coating buffers. The coated plate should be used freshly.

2. Coating and incubating should be carried out in a humidified box.

[Question]

Why can you use one enzyme-labelled second-antibody to check many pairs of antigen and antibody?

(Zhang Xiaolian)

实验三十六 间接免疫荧光法

【原理】

间接免疫荧光法是用荧光素标记的二抗检测 Ag 或 Ab 的一种实验技术。其原理是 Ag 首先与一抗结合,然后一抗再与荧光素标记的二抗结合,形成一个 Ag－Ab_1-荧光素标记 Ab_2 的三分子复合物,在荧光显微镜下呈现荧光。

【用途】

下面以检测 T 淋巴细胞亚群为例介绍间接免疫荧光法。

【材料】

1. 肝素抗凝血
2. 淋巴细胞分离液:密度(1.077±0.001) g/L
3. 鼠抗人 T 淋巴细胞 McAb(Ab_1):抗 CD_3、抗 CD_4、抗 CD_8
4. 荧光标记羊抗鼠 IgG(Ab_2)
5. 含 5%胎牛血清的 Hank's 液
6. EP 管、试管、吸管、载玻片、盖玻片、离心机、荧光显微镜等

【方法】

1. 取肝素抗凝血 2 mL,分离淋巴细胞,用含 5%胎牛血清的 Hank's 液配成 $1.5×10^6$ 个/mL 的淋巴细胞悬液。
2. 取 4 个 EP 管,每管加 100 μL 淋巴细胞分离液,3 000 r/min 离心 10 min。
3. 弃上清,每管加 CD_3、CD_4、CD_8 的 McAb 各 25 μL(1∶25 稀释),对照管加 Hank's 液 25 μL。混匀,4℃作用 30 min。

$1^\#$管 — CD_3 McAb

$2^\#$管 — CD_4 McAb

$3^\#$管 — CD_8 McAb

$4^\#$管 —含 5% FCS 的 Hank's 液(对照管)

4. 用含 5%胎牛血清的 Hank's 液离洗 3 次,每次 1 500 r/min 离心 10 min。
5. 弃上清,每管加 1∶20 荧光标记羊抗鼠 IgG 50 μL,混匀,4℃避光作用 30 min。
6. 含 5%胎牛血清的用 Hank's 液离洗 3 次,每次 1 500 r/min 离心 10 min。
7. 弃上清,每管加 20 μL 含 5%胎牛血清的 Hank's 液,混匀,取一滴细胞悬液于载玻片,加盖玻片,荧光显微镜下观察。

【结果】

在荧光显微镜下,细胞膜上发荧光的为阳性细胞。计数 200 个淋巴细胞,计算出各 T

淋巴细胞亚群的百分率。

T 淋巴细胞亚群参考值为：CD_3^+ T 70% ~ 80%、CD_4^+ T 40% ~ 60%、CD_8^+ T 20% ~ 30%。

【注意事项】

1. 荧光标记的抗体应置 4℃冰箱中保存，避免反复冻融，使用前新鲜配制。
2. 荧光染色后一般在 1 h 内完成实验，时间过长，会使荧光减弱。
3. 各 T 淋巴细胞亚群的正常范围随各实验室的实验方法、条件的不同稍有差异。

【思考题】

为什么用间接免疫荧光法可检测 T 淋巴细胞亚群？

（刘　春）

Exp. 36   Indirect Immunofluorescence Assay

【Principle】

Indirect immunofluorescence assay is the technique that detects unknown antigen or antibody by secondary antibody-fluorochrome. Antigen is combined first with unlabelled primary antibody, followed combined with secondary antibody-fluorochrome and a three molecular complex consisting of antigen, antibody and secondary antibody-fluorochrome is formed. It will appear fluorescence under fluorescent microscope.

【Application】

Here is an example of indirect immunofluorescence assay for detecting T lymphocyte subset.

【Materials】

1. Heparinized blood

2. Lymphocyte separation medium: specific gravity (1.077 ± 0.001) g/L

3. Mouse antihuman monoclonal antibody (Ab_1): anti-CD_3, anti-CD_4, anti-CD_8

4. Fluorochrome labelled goat anti-mouse IgG (Ab_2)

5. HBSS containing 5% fetal calf serum

6. Test tube, eppendorf tube, pipette, centrifuge tube, centrifuge, fluorescent microscope, slide, cover glass, etc.

【Procedures】

1. Take 2 mL heparinied blood and separate lymphocyte. Adjust cell suspension to 1.5×10^6 cells/mL using HBSS containing 5% fetal calf serum.

2. Mark four eppendorf tubes 1 to 4. Add 100 μL of lymphocyte suspension into each eppendorf tube. Centrifuge at 3,000 r/min for 10 min.

3. Discard the supernatant. Add 25 μL (1 : 25 dilution) of mouse anti-human monoclonal antibody into the corresponding tube:

Tube 1 — CD_3 McAb

Tube 2 — CD_4 McAb

Tube 3 — CD_8 McAb

Tube 4 — HBSS containing 5% FCS (control tube)

Mix well. Place at 4℃ for 30 min.

4. Wash three times with HBSS containing 5% fetal calf serum by centrifugation at 1,500 r/min for 10 min.

5. Decant the supernatant. Add 50 μL of 1 : 20 fluorochrome labeled goat anti-mouse IgG. Mix well. Place in 4℃ in the dark for 30 min.

6. Wash three times with HBSS containing 5% fetal calf serum by centrifugation at 1,500 r/min for 10 min.

7. Discard the supernatant. Add 20 μL of HBSS containing 5% fetal calf serum. Mix well. Take a drop of cell suspension to the slide and put a cover glass. Read fluorescence under a fluorescent microscope.

【Results】

Indirect immunofluorescence assay may be read manually with a fluorescent microscope. Positive cells mean the T lymphocytes with fluorescence on the cell surface membrane. Count 200 viable lymphocytes and calculate the percentage of T lymphocyte subset.

T lymphocyte subset reference value: CD_3^+ T 70%−80%, CD_4^+ T 40%−60%, CD_8^+ T 20%−30%.

【Precautions】

1. Fluorochrome labelled antibody must be stored at 4℃. Do not freeze before using.

2. Indirect immunofluorescence assay results are read generally within an hour. If the time is too long, fluorescence becomes weaker and weaker.

3. Reference ranges of T lymphocyte subset must be developed by each laboratory.

【Question】

Why can T lymphocyte subsets be detected by indirect immunofluorescence assay?

(Liu Chun)

实验三十七　　免疫胶体金技术——测定 HBsAg 的试纸条双抗体夹心法

【原理】

免疫胶体金技术（ICGT）是以胶体金作为标志物检测抗原—抗体反应的一种免疫标记检测技术。胶体金是氯金酸（$HAuCl_4$）在还原剂作用下聚合而成的颗粒，然后在静电作用下形成稳定的胶体状态，故称为胶体金。胶体金颗粒在弱碱环境下带负电荷，可与免疫球蛋白、抗原等生物大分子牢固结合，又不影响生物大分子的生物学特性，是可以应用于免疫反应的优良标记物。根据胶体金的一些物理性状，如高电子密度、颗粒大小及颜色反应，通过肉眼或仪器判定，可定性定量检测血液、尿液、体液等样本中的抗原或抗体的有无或者多少。

本实验是试纸条双抗体夹心法免疫胶体金技术检测血液样本中 HBsAg，其原理是：在胶体金结合垫上含有胶体金标记的 HBsAg 抗体（金标 Ab_1），检测线（T 线）中含有 HBsAg 抗体（Ab_1），质控线（C 线）中含有羊抗鼠 IgG（Ab_2）。将待检样本加到试纸条一端的样本垫上后，样本在硝酸纤维素膜上通过毛细作用、层析作用，慢慢向另一端渗移。若样本中含有 HBsAg，即阳性样本，HBsAg 将与胶体金垫上的金标 Ab_1 反应，形成抗原—金标抗体复合物；当样本移动至检测线时，会与包被的 Ab_1 形成抗原—抗体—金标抗体复合物，在 T 线位置呈现出红色条带。若样本中无 HBsAg，则不能形成复合物，T 线位置上不出现红色条带。当液相继续迁移至 C 线，会与包被的 Ab_2 结合，在检测样本时 C 线位置均应出现红色条带（图 37−1）。

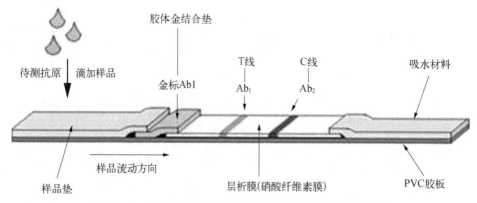

图 37−1　试纸条双抗体夹心法免疫层析胶体金技术示意图

【应用】

常用的有免疫胶体金光镜染色法、免疫胶体金电镜染色法、斑点金免疫渗滤法及基于胶体金免疫层析法，研发的各种诊断试纸条，用于抗原及抗体的便捷、快速检测。

【材料】

1. 血清或血浆样本
2. HBsAg 胶体金法检测试剂盒
3. 一次性塑料吸管

【方法】

1. 条型试剂：

（1）将检测试剂及样本平衡至 25～30℃，撕开铝箔袋，取出检测试纸。

（2）在试纸的加样端加入约 80 μL 血清或血浆，或将试纸的加样端插入待检样本中（注意不要超过 MAX 线）3～10 s，等样本开始在层析膜上时取出，平放。

（3）用计时器计时，30 min 内观察实验结果，超过 40 min 则结果无效。

2. 卡型试剂：

（1）将检测试剂及样本平衡至 25～30℃，撕开铝箔袋，取出检测卡，平放。

（2）用滴管吸取样本，在检测卡的加样孔加入约 3 滴（约 90 μL）血清或血浆。

（3）用计时器计时，30 min 内观察实验结果，超过 40 min 则结果无效。

【结果】

阳性（+）：质控线（C 线）和检测线（T 线）出现二条红色条带。

阴性（-）：仅在质控线（C 线）出现一条红色条带。

无效：质控线（C 线）不出现红色条带或仅检测线（T 线）出现一条红色条带，结果无效，应重试。

【注意事项】

1. 血清或血浆标本可于 4℃保存 48 h，在-30℃下冻存 6 个月。冷冻标本检测前应充分融化、摇匀，并恢复至 25～30℃。

2. 试剂盒从包装袋内取出，应在撕口后 1 h 内使用，尽可能即开即用。

3. 质控线（C 线）红色条带的出现表明操作步骤及方法是正确的，质控线无红色条带出现，提示操作不当：如样本量不够，层析过程不正常或试剂盒已过效期或试剂盒已经损坏。

【思考题】

1. 如何用试纸条双抗体夹心法免疫层析胶体金技术诊断早期妊娠？
2. 请设计检测 HIV 抗体的免疫胶体金试纸条。

（王　瑾）

HBsAg Test Trip by Double Antigen Sandwich Immune Colloidal Gold Strip Technique

【Principle】

Immune colloidal gold technique (ICT) is an immunolabelling technique which has been widely applied for antigen-antibody detection. Colloidal gold is a particle formed by the polymerization of chloroauric acid (HAuCl$_4$) under the action of a reducing agent, and then forms a stable colloidal state under the action of static electricity, so it is called colloidal gold. Colloidal gold particles are negatively charged in a weak alkaline environment and can be attached to many traditional biological probes such as immunoglobulins and antigens without affecting the biological properties of biological macromolecules. Thus becoming an excellent marker that can be applied for immune responses detecting. According to some physical properties of colloidal gold, such as high electron density, particle size, and color reaction, we can qualitatively and quantitatively detect the presence or absence of antigen or antibody in blood, urine, body fluid and other samples.

HBsAg test strip (double-antibody sandwich immunochromatography colloidal gold technology) This experiment is a double-antibody sandwich immunochromatography colloidal gold technique for detecting HBsAg in blood samples. The principle is as follows.

HBsAg test is an antibody sandwich immunoassay. Colloidal gold conjugated monoclonal antibodies reactive to HBsAg (gold-Ab$_1$) are dry-immobilized onto a nitrocellulose membrane strip. When the sample is added, it migrates by capillary diffusion through the strip rehydrating the gold conjugate. If present, HBsAg will bind with the gold conjugated antibodies forming particles. These particles will continue to migrate along the strip until the Test Zone (T line) where they are captured by antiHBs antibodies (Ab$_1$) immobilized there and a visible red line appears. If there is no HBsAg in sample, no red line will appear in the Test Zone (T line). The gold conjugate will continue to migrate alone until is captured in the Control Zone (C line) from immobilized goat anti-mouse IgG antibody (Ab$_2$) and aggregated in a red line, which indicates the validity of the test (Fig.37 − 1).

【Applications】

Immunocolloidal gold light microscopy, immunocolloidal gold electron microscopy, dot gold immunofiltration, and colloidal gold immunochromatography

【Materials】

1. Serum or plasma specimen

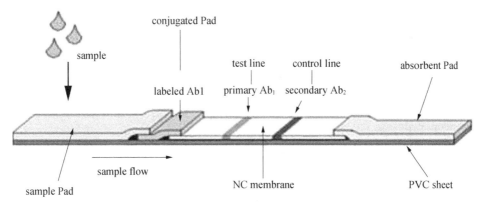

Fig.37 - 1   Sketch map of double-antibody sandwich immunochromatography colloidal gold technology

2. HBsAg kit (colloidal gold)

3. Disposable sample dropper

【Procedures】

1. Strip reagent:

(1) Remove the test device from the foil pouch, and place it on a flat, dry surface.

(2) Add about 80 μL of serum into the sampling end of the test strip with a disposable dropper, or insert the sample end of the test strip into the sample to be tested (be careful not to exceed the MAX line) 3 - 10 seconds, and then take it out when the sample starts on the chromatographic membrane.

(3) Read the results within 30 min. If it is over 40 min, the result will be invalid.

2. Card type reagent:

(1) Remove the testing device from the foil pouch by tearing at the "notch". Then place the testing device on a level surface.

(2) Hold the Sample Dropper vertically, add three drops (90 μL) of specimen without air bubbles into the sample well marked with an arrow on the testing device.

(3) Read the results within 30 min. If it is over 40 min, the result will be invalid.

【Results】

Positive (+): two pink color bands appear at the control and test line regions.

Negative (-): only one pink color band appears on the control region (C line).

Invalid: no visible band at control region or only a pink band appears on the test line (T line). Repeat with a new test device.

【Precautions】

1. Serum or plasma samples can be stored at 4℃ for 48 hours and frozen at -30℃ for 6 months. Frozen specimens should be fully thawed, shaken, and returned to room temperature

(25 - 30℃) before testing.

2. The kit should be used within 1 hour or immediately after removing from the pouch.

3. The appearance of the red line of the quality control line (C line) indicates the steps and methods. There is no red band on the quality control line, which suggests failure of test. Such as: insufficient sample size, abnormal chromatographic process or expired kit or the kit has been damaged.

【Questions】

1. How to diagnose early pregnancy with double-antibody sandwich immunochromatography colloidal gold technology?

2. Design an immunocolloidal gold test strip for the detection of HIV antibodies.

(Ma Yunfeng　Ji Yanhong)

实验三十八　化学发光免疫标记技术检测乳腺癌患者 HER-2 胞外结构域（ECD）

【原理】

化学发光免疫标记技术(CLIA)是将具有高灵敏度的化学发光测定技术与高特异性的免疫反应相结合,在组织、细胞及分子水平对抗原—抗体反应进行直接观察或自动化测定的检测方法。

该方法以化学发光剂、催化发光酶或产物间接参与发光反应的物质等标记抗体或抗原,当标记抗体或标记抗原与相应抗原或抗体结合后,发光底物受发光剂、催化酶或参与产物作用,生成激发态中间体,当回复至稳定的基态时发射光子,通过发光分析仪测定光子产量,进行待检样品中抗体或抗原测定。

化学发光免疫标记技术根据化学发光所用的标记物和发光原理的不同可分为三类:化学发光免疫标记技术(CLIA)、化学发光酶免疫标记技术(CLEIA)和电化学发光免疫标记技术(ECLIA)。

化学发光免疫标记技术(CLIA)是将化学发光剂(如吖啶酯、鲁米诺等)标记抗原或抗体。主要是通过激发发光试剂 $NaOH+H_2O_2$ 作用而发光。其中小分子物质的检测多采用竞争法,大分子物质的检测主要用夹心法(图 38-1)。

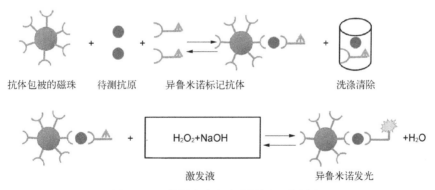

抗体包被的磁珠　　待测抗原　　异鲁米诺标记抗体　　　　　　洗涤清除

激发液　　　　　　异鲁米诺发光　　+H₂O

图 38-1　化学发光免疫分析标记示意图

化学发光酶免疫标记技术(CLEIA)是用催化某一化学发光反应的酶来标记抗原或抗体,发生抗原抗体特异性反应后,形成固相包被抗体—待测抗原—酶标记抗体复合物;当加入发光剂试剂后,酶催化和分解底物发光(图 38-2);测定发光体系的发光强度即可对抗体或抗原进行定性或定量测定。

电化学发光免疫标记技术(ECLIA)源于电化学法和化学发光法,是一种在电极表面由电化学引发的特异性化学发光反应,包括电化学和化学发光两个过程。即以电化学发光剂三联吡啶钌($[Rb(bpy)_3]^{2+}$)标记抗原或抗体,以三丙胺(TPA)为电子供体,在电场中因电子转移而发生特异性化学发光反应(图 38-3,图 38-4)。

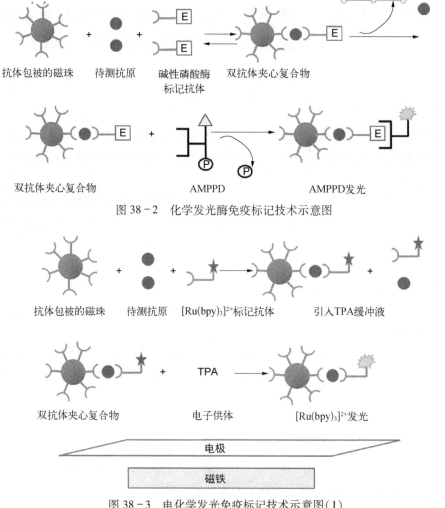

图 38-2　化学发光酶免疫标记技术示意图

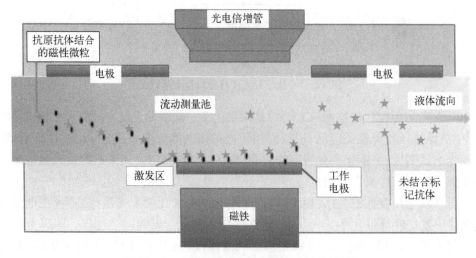

图 38-3　电化学发光免疫标记技术示意图(1)

图 38-4　电化学发光免疫标记技术示意图(2)

20% ~ 30% 乳腺癌患者过表达人类表皮生长因子受体 2(HER－2)。HER－2 为分子量 185 000 Da、具有酪氨酸激酶活性的跨膜蛋白,由胞外结构域(ECD)、跨膜结构域和细胞内结构域 3 部分组成,其中 ECD 可被降解释放到外周血中并被检测到,ECD 过表达与肿瘤的发生、发展和预后关系密切,ECD 检测为乳腺癌患者的诊断、治疗、评价和判断预后提供依据。

【应用】

该技术具有光信号持续时间长、灵敏度高、分析方法简便快速、标记效率高、安全稳定、可实现自动化分析、本底低等优点,广泛用于各种抗原、半抗原、抗体、激素、酶、脂肪酸、维生素和药物等超微量活性物质的检测分析技术。此外,临床上可以用于化学发光免疫分析检测肿瘤标志物,例如甲胎蛋白(AFP)、癌胚抗原(CEA)、糖类抗原(CA125、CA153、CA199)、前列腺特异抗原(PSA)、鳞状细胞癌抗原(SCC)、磷脂酰肌醇蛋白聚糖(GPC3)、P53 蛋白等。

本实验应用 CILA 技术检测乳腺癌患者 HER－2 的 CD 表达。

【材料】

1. 临床血清样本
2. HER－2 ECD 测定试剂盒,主要成分包括:吖啶酯标记的鼠抗人单克隆抗体 TA－1,荧光素标记的鼠抗人单克隆抗体 NB－3,重组表达的 HER－2 ECD 标准品
3. 洗板仪
4. 全自动免疫发光分析仪

【步骤】

1. 将待检样本加入包被有鼠单克隆抗体的包被珠,分别使用吖啶酯标记的鼠抗人单克隆抗体 TA－1 和荧光素标记的鼠抗人单克隆抗体 NB－3 与 HER－2 ECD 上的抗原决定簇特异性结合,形成免疫复合物并激发化学发光反应。
2. 确保室内质控品检测结果均在正常范围。
3. 全自动免疫分析仪读板。

【结果】

样品的相对吸光值与其中的 HER－2 ECD 浓度呈正相关。样品中的 HER－2 ECD 浓度依据由标准品 HER－2 ECD 浓度和对应的 RLU 建立的数学模型进行定量。结果采用 SPSS 18.0 软件进行统计分析。HER－2 ECD>15.2 ng/mL 为阳性。

【注意事项】

1. 血清标本不宜反复冻融,4℃保存时间不超过一周。
2. 试剂盒 2~8℃避光保存,应在有效期内使用。

【思考题】

请比较酶标记技术与化学发光技术的特点。

（韩　莉）

Exp. 38   Detection of HER−2 Extracellular Domain of Breast Cancer Patients by Chemiluminescence Immunoassay

【Principle】

Chemiluminescence immunoassay (CLIA) is a detection method that combines highly sensitive chemiluminescence technique with highly specific immunochemical reactions. CLIA is based on labelled antibodies or antigens with chemiluminescence agents, catalytic luminescent enzymes or products, and the luminescence reaction indirectly. It has been used to directly observe or automatically test the antigen-antibody reactions of tissues, cells and molecules. When the labelled antibody or labelled antigen binds to the antigen or antibody speicficly, the luminescent substrate is activated by the luminescent agent, catalytic enzyme or participating product to form an excited intermediate active state. Then the activated intermediates emit photon during their return to the stable ground state. The amount of the antibody or antigen in the sample can be determined by detecting the photon yield with a luminescence analyzer.

According to the different labelling material used, the method has three types: chemiluminescence immunoassay (CLIA), chemiluminescence enzyme immunoassay (CLEIA) and electrochemiluminescence immunoassay (ECLIA).

For chemiluminescence immunoassay (CLIA), the antigens or antibodies are labelled by chemiluminescent agents (such as acridinium ester, luminol, etc.), which can be illuminated by NaOH and H_2O_2. The competitive method is used for the micromolecular substance detecting, and the sandwich method is used for the macromolecular substance detection as shown in Fig.38−1.

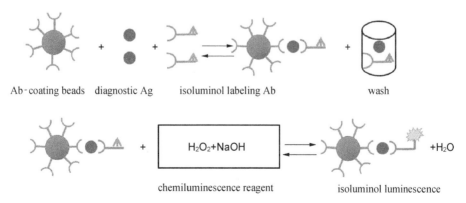

Fig.38−1   Schematic diagram of chemiluminescence immunoassay

For chemiluminescent enzyme immunoassay (CLEIA), the antigens or antibodies are labelled by an enzyme that specifically catalyzes the chemiluminescence reaction. After the immune reaction they form a complex, including solid phase coated antibody — antigen to be tested and enzyme labelled antibody, then the chemiluminescence reagents are added. Enzyme catalyzes and decomposes the substrate to emit light (Fig. 38 − 2). The amount antibody or antigen is determined by measuring the luminescence intensity of the luminescence reaction.

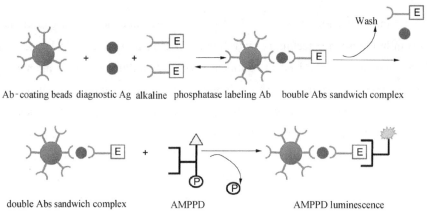

Fig.38 − 2　Schematic diagram of chemiluminescent enzyme immunoassay

Electrochemiluminescence immunoassay (ECLIA) is a chemiluminescence reaction initiated by electrochemistry on the electrode surface. It combinates electrochemical and chemiluminescence methods, which consists of electrochemistry and chemiluminescence processes. The antigens or antibodies are labelled by the electrochemical luminescent reagents such as triple pyridinium ($[Rb(bpy)_3]^{2+}$) and the electron donor is tripropylamine (TPA). The chemiluminescence reaction arises from an electron transfer in an electric field as shown in Fig.38 − 3 and Fig.38 − 4.

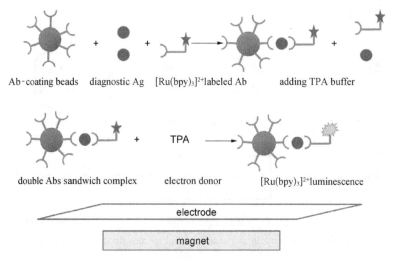

Fig.38 − 3　Diagram of electrochemiluminescence immunoassay reaction

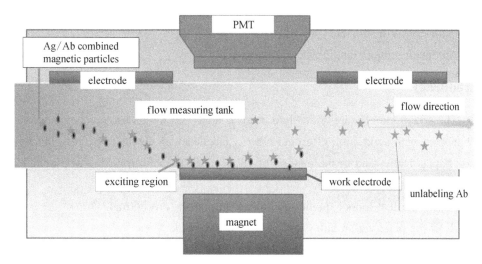

Fig.38−4　Diagram of electrochemiluminescence immunoassay working pricinple

Human epidermal growth factor receptor 2 (HER−2) is overexpressed in 20% to 30% of breast cancer patients. HER−2 is a transmembrane protein with 185,000 Da which has tyrosine kinase activity. HER−2 consists of extracellular domain (ECD), transmembrane domain and intracellular domain. ECD can be degraded and released into peripheral blood, thus it can be detected in the serum. ECD overexpression is closely related to the occurrence, development and prognosis of tumors. ECD detection provides a basis for the diagnosis, treatment, evaluation and prognosis of breast cancer patients.

【Application】

The technology has the advantages of long duration of optical signal, high sensitivity, simple and rapid analysis, high marking efficiency, safety and stability, automatic analysis and low background. Chemoluminescence immunoassay can be applied in the detection and analysis of super tiny amount of various antigens, haptens, antibodies, hormones, enzymes, fatty acids, vitamins and drugs, etc. It can also be used to detect tumor markers of alpha-fetoprotein (AFP), carcinoembryonic antigen (CEA), carbohydrate antigens (CA125, CA153, CA199), prostate specific antigen (PSA), squamous cell carcinoma antigen (SCC), phosphatidylinositol (GPC3), P53 protein, and so on.

In this experiment, human epidermal growth factor receptor 2 (HER−2) extracellular domain (ECD) of breast cancer patients is detected by CILA.

【Materials】

1. Clinical serum samples

2. HER−2 ECD assay kit with mouse monoclonal antibody TA − 1 labeled acridinium ester, mouse monoclonal antibody NB −3 labeled fluorescein, and the standards of

recombinant HER－2 ECD

   3. Plate-rinsing instrument

   4. Automatic immunoluminescence analyzer

【Procedures】

1. The serum samples are added into beads coated with the mouse monoclonal antibodies TA－1 labeled with acridinium ester and NB－3 labelled with fluorescein, respectively. The antibodies specifically bind to the epitope of HER－2 ECD to form an immune complex and elicit a chemiluminescent reaction.

2. Make sure that indoor quality control testing results are normal.

3. Read the plate via an automated immunoassay reader.

【Results】

The relative light unit (RLU) of the sample is positively correlated with the concentration of HER－2 ECD. The HER－2 ECD concentration in the sample is determined by a mathematical model established from the concentrations of HER－2 ECD and the corresponding RLU in a standards. The data is analyzed by software SPSS version 18.0. The results are positive when the concentration of HER－2 ECD above 15.2 ng/mL.

【Precautions】

1. Serum samples should be stored at 4℃ for less than one week and can not be frozen and thawed repeatedly.

2. The kit should be stored at 2－8℃ in the dark and used in validity date.

【Question】

Please compare the characteristics of enzyme labelling technique with chemiluminescence technique.

(Han Li)

实验三十九　　生物发光技术

【原理】

生物发光是生物体内一种由特定酶催化,将生物化学能转化为光能的化学发光现象。生物发光技术通过将荧光素酶基因整合到预期观察的细胞染色体 DNA 中以表达荧光素酶,然后培养出能稳定表达荧光素酶的细胞株。将标记好的细胞接种到实验动物体内后,当外源(腹腔或静脉注射)给予其底物荧光素(luciferin),在生物体内环境中三磷酸腺苷(ATP)、O_2 及 Mg^{2+} 存在的条件下,荧光素酶催化底物荧光素发生氧化脱羧反应,释放可见光能,从而实现生物发光(偏红色),通过电荷耦合器件(CCD)设备等生物光学成像系统进行检测,即生物发光活体成像(BLI)技术。基因、细胞和活体动物都可被荧光素酶基因标记。荧光素酶在标记细胞内的表达可以直接指示细胞在体内的活动和反应,其中 ATP提供生化反应所需的能量,即该反应必须在活细胞内才会存在和产生发光现象,且发光强度与标记细胞的数目线性相关(发光原理如图 39-1 所示)。

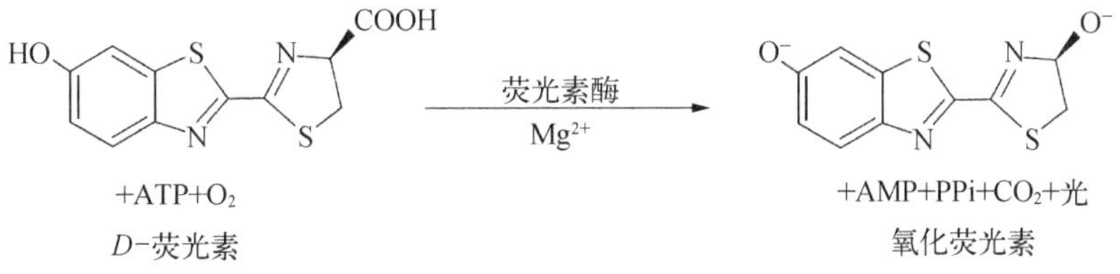

图 39-1　萤火虫荧光素酶的发光原理

这种无需激发光就可发出的生物荧光,组织穿透能力强,灵敏度高,由于没有激发光的非特异性干扰,信噪比较高。

【应用】

生物发光技术因具有极高的灵敏度,便于对疾病动物模型微小病灶进行检测,而且不涉及放射性有害物质,安全系数高,实验结果直观,可精确定量,重现性好,操作简便,得到迅速发展。目前该技术已应用于医疗卫生、食品、环境等领域,尤其在抗肿瘤研究领域应用极为广泛,实现了在活体内实时、连续地对肿瘤细胞生长、浸润、转移等恶性生物学行为的检测,也可进行药物选择及个体化治疗。

【材料】

以裸鼠肺腺癌模型检测为例:

(1) 雄性裸鼠(6~8 周龄)

(2) 单克隆抗体 NJ001(特异性识别肺腺癌及其他非小细胞肺癌细胞中的 SP70抗原)

（3）750 nm 磁珠

（4）人肺腺癌细胞株 SPC－A1－luc(稳定表达荧光素酶)，荧光素

（5）RPMI－1640 培养液、胎牛血清、羊血清工作液

（6）小动物可见光活体成像系统，小动物活体 micro-CT 影像系统

【方法】

1. NJ001 免疫磁珠的制备：

（1）采用 EDC/NHS 法将磁珠与单抗 NJ001 偶联。取 1 mg 磁珠用 500 μL MEST (10 mmol/L MES，0.5‰吐温-20，pH 6.0) 洗涤 3 次。400 μL MES (10 mmol/L，pH 6.0) 重悬磁珠后加入 0.5 mg EDC，0.5 mg NHS，置于混匀仪上保持悬浮状态，37℃活化 1 h。

（2）磁分离去上清，500 μL MEST 洗涤 2 次，PBST (0.01 mol/L PBS，0.1‰吐温-20，pH 7.4) 重悬后加入 NJ001 抗体 250 μg (50 μL×5 μg/mL)，于 4℃过夜混匀。

（3）偶联产物与乙醇胺(2%，V/V) 37℃ 混匀 1 h。

（4）PBST 洗涤 3 次后加 1 mL PBST (含 0.5% BSA，0.02% NaN₃) 重悬，4℃保存。

（5）将上述制备的免疫磁珠调整到合适浓度注射小鼠。

2. 细胞培养及裸鼠肺腺癌模型的建立：

（1）SPC－A1－luc 细胞生长于含有 10%胎牛血清的 RPMI－1640 培养液，在 37℃、5%CO_2培养箱中传代培养。

（2）取对数生长期的细胞 PBS 洗涤后调整细胞浓度为 $5×10^6$个/mL，尾静脉注射 100 μL 细胞悬液(裸鼠饲养于 SPF 级环境中，26~28℃，湿度 40%~60%，所用垫料、饮水、标准饲料及其他与实验动物接触的物品均经高压蒸汽灭菌处理)。

3. 肺癌裸鼠的干预：

（1）肺腺癌裸鼠模型随机分为生理盐水组、裸磁珠组和免疫磁珠组。

（2）每周通过尾静脉分别注射相应的溶液：生理盐水组每只注射生理盐水 100 μL，裸磁珠组注射 1∶50 稀释的 750 nm 磁珠悬液 100 μL，免疫磁珠组注射 1∶50 稀释的偶联 NJ001 的 750 nm 磁珠溶液 100 μL。

（3）每周注射前和注射后 4 h 分别进行 micro-CT 扫描。

4. 小动物可见光活体成像检测：

（1）每周利用生物发光成像系统检测肺部肿瘤生物发光信号值，监测肺部肿瘤的生长。

（2）检测时每只裸鼠按 150 mg/kg 的量腹腔注射荧光素底物，异氟烷麻醉后 10~15 min 进行活体成像，成像后应用系统自带软件检测肺部肿瘤生物发光信号强度。

（3）实验数据采用 GraphPad Prism 6.0 软件进行统计分析。

【结果】

裸鼠尾静脉接种 SPC－A1－luc 细胞后，每周注射底物荧光素进行生物发光成像。肺部生物发光信号由弥散分布逐渐聚集于裸鼠肺部，且第 2 周开始裸鼠肺部生物发光信号随时间延长而升高，可见肺部已经形成实体瘤。生理盐水组和裸磁珠组在第 4 周就可以

检测到肿瘤,并且随着时间延长肿瘤不断增大,免疫磁珠组到第 6 周才检测到肿瘤。

【注意事项】

由于荧光素酶的活性和稳定性受很多因素影响,如缓冲液种类、温度、pH、金属离子、酶浓度及发光测定时间等,尤其 pH 对其影响最大,在使用中需要加以注意。

【思考题】

1. 试比较生物发光技术与化学发光技术的优缺点。
2. 哪些因素可影响荧光素酶的活性?

（周永芹）

【Principle】

Bioluminescence is a chemiluminescence phenomenon catalyzed by a specific enzyme *in vivo*, which converts biochemical energy into optical energy. The bioluminescence assay is performed through integrating the gene of luciferase into the chromosome DNA of cells expected to be observed. Then the cells with positively and stably luciferase expression are screened out. After inoculating the labelled cells into the experimental animals and exogenous administration (intraperitoneal or intravascular injecting) of the substrate luciferin, luciferase catalyzes the oxidative decarboxylation reaction of luciferin under the presence of adenosine triphosphate (ATP), oxygen (O_2) and magnesium (Mg^{2+}), and then emits visible light and enables bioluminescence (reddish). The light is detected by bioluminescence imaging system such as charge coupled device (CCD), which is so called the bioluminescence imaging (BLI). Genes, cells and living animals can be labelled by the luciferase gene. The luciferase expressed in the labelled cells can directly indicate the activities and reactions of the labeled cells *in vivo*. ATP provides the energy needed for biochemical reactions, which means that the bioluminescence only exists and can be detected within living cells, moreover, the luminous intensity is linearly correlated with the amount of the cells labelled (the principle of luminescence is shown on Fig.39 − 1).

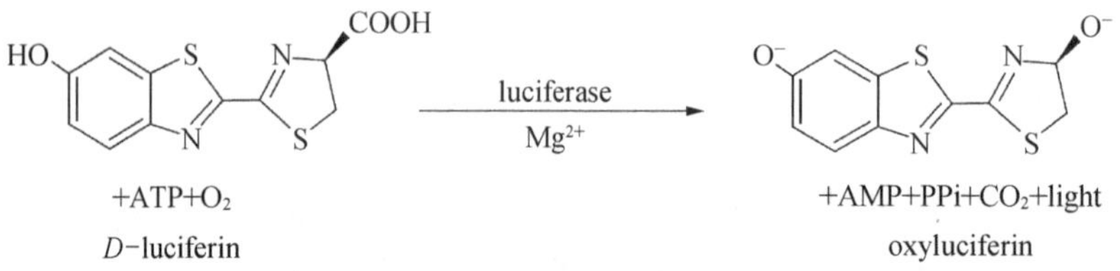

Fig.39 − 1   The mechanism of luminescence by firefly luciferase

The bioluminescence is emitted independent of the exciting light, and it has strong tissue penetration, high sensitivity, and high signal-to-noise ratio as lacking the non-specific interference of exciting light.

【Application】

The bioluminescence assay is easy to be used in detecting the tiny nidus in animal models of disease due to its high sensitivity and safety, non-radioactive materials. The result of the bioluminescence assay is intuitive, and can be accurately quantified with fine reproducibility, and simple operation, etc. Nowadays this technique is widely used in health care, food, and environment, especially in the field of anti-tumor research. The bioluminescence assay can be timely and consecutively used to monitor the growth, invasion and metastasis of malignant tumor, or select drugs and individualized treatment.

【Materials】

Detection of lung adenocarcinoma in nude mouse model with lung cancer is used as an example:

(1) male nude mice (6 – 8 weeks old)

(2) monoclonal antibody for NJ001 (which can specifically recognize the antigen SP70 of the lung adenocarcinoma cells and other non-small cell lung cancer cells)

(3) 750 nm magnetic bead

(4) SPC – A1 – luc cell line (with stable expression of luciferase), luciferin

(5) RPMI – 1640 medium, fetal bovine serum, sheep serum working solution

(6) Small animal visible light living imaging system, small animal living micro-CT imaging system

【Procedures】

1. Preparation of NJ001 immunomagnetic beads:

(1) Combine the magnetic beads with the monoantibody NJ001 through the method of EDC/NHS. First, 1 mg beads are washed with 500 μL MEST (10 mmol/L MES, 0.5‰ Tween 20, pH 6.0) for 3 times and resuspended with 400 μL MES (10 mmol/L, pH 6.0)

0.5 mg EDC and 0.5 mg NHS are added into the MES. Keep the suspension status of beads to active for 1 h on a shaker at 37℃.

(2) Separate Magnetic and discard the supernatant, then wash the magnetic beads with 500 μL MEST twice, resuspended with PBST (0.01mol/L PBS, 0.1‰ Tween 20, pH 7.4)

Add 250 μg of antibody NJ001 (50 μL×5 μg/mL) overnight at 4 ℃.

(3) Mix immunomagnetic beads and 2% ethanolamine (V/V) for 1h, wash with PBST for 3 times, then add 1 mL PBST (containing 0.5% BSA, 0.02% NaN3) to resuspend and store at 4℃.

(4) Dilute the prepared immunomagnetic beads to proper concentration for injecting into mouse.

2. Cell culture and induction of lung adenocarcinoma in nude mice:

(1) SPC – A1 – luc cells are cultured by RPMI – 1640 medium with 10% fetal bovine serum in a incubator with 5% CO_2 at 37 ℃.

(2) Harvest the cells at logarithmic phase, wash with PBS and then adjust the concentration to $5×10^6$ cells/mL.

Tail vein injection of 100 μL SPC – A1 – luc cell suspension into nude mouse (nude mice are housed in the SPF conditions with 26 – 28℃, 40%－60% humidity. The bedding, drinking water, standard feed and other materials in contact with the experiment animals are processed by high pressure steam sterilization).

3. Intervention of lung adenocarcinoma nude mice:

(1) The lung adenocarcinoma nude mice are randomly divided into 3 groups: physiological saline group, bare bead group and immunomagnetic bead group.

(2) The following solution is injected through tail vein once a week: 100 μL of physiological saline per mouse for physiological saline group, 100 μL of 750 nm bare bead (1 : 50 diluted) per mouse for bare bead group and 100 μL of immunomagenetic bead coupled with antibody NJ001 (1 : 50 diluted) per mouse for immunomagnetic bead group.

(3) Scan the mouse with micro-CT 4 h before and after the injection every week.

4. Detecting the lung tumor with small animal visible light living imaging system:

(1) The bioluminescence signal intensity of lung tumor is detected by a bioluminescence imaging system to monitor the growth of lung tumor every week.

(2) During the detection the nude mice are intraperitoneally injected with 150 mg/kg of luciferin substrate and imagined after anesthesia by isoflurane for 10 - 15 min, then the bioluminescence signal intensity of lung tumor is analyzed by the software.

(3) Statistical analysis is performed by GraphPad Prism 6.0.

【Results】

Following SPC - A1 - luc cells being inoculated into the tail vein of nude mice, the substrate luciferin was injected for bioluminescence imaging weekly. The bioluminescence signal gradually is gathered from the dispersed distribution to the lungs of nude mice. From the second week the bioluminescence signal intensity is increased with the prolongation of time in the lung of nude mice, which indicating the formation of solid tumors in the lung. The tumors were detected in normal saline group and naked magnetic beads group in the fourth week, and it grows continuously over time. While the tumor can be detected in the immunomagnetic beads group until the sixth week.

【Precautions】

Because the activity and stability of luciferase are affected by many factors, such as buffer, temperature, pH, metal ions, enzyme concentration and luminescence detecting time, etc. pH change has the greatest influence on it, so it needs more attention to pH value.

【Questions】

1. Compare the advantages and disadvantages of bioluminescence technology and chemiluminescence technology.

2. What factors may influence the activity of luciferase?

(Zhou Yongqin)

第七篇
Chapter Seven

细胞凋亡的检测技术和流式细胞术
Flow Cytometry and Cell Apoptosis Detection Technique

实验四十　　细胞凋亡的 DNA 琼脂糖凝胶电泳分析

【原理】

细胞凋亡是机体生长发育中细胞自主性死亡的过程。细胞凋亡过程中有一系列特征性的形态学改变。其中最重要和最具有特征性的改变是 Ca^{2+}/Mg^{2+} 依赖性的核酸内切酶的激活导致染色质 DNA 在核小体连接部位断裂,形成以 $180\sim200$ bp 为最小单位的单体或寡聚体片段。检测细胞凋亡的常用方法有流式细胞术法,DNA 琼脂糖凝胶电泳,DNA 3′端标记以后再进行凝胶电泳和放射自显影,以及末端转移酶介导的缺口末端标记(TUNEL)等方法。

DNA 琼脂糖凝胶电泳是最早用于研究细胞凋亡生物化学变化特性的传统方法。DNA 琼脂糖凝胶电泳是检测细胞凋亡过程中 DNA 降解的敏感、特异、快速的方法,随着核酸内切酶的活化,DNA 降解成寡核小体,这些降解片段均为 $180\sim200$ bp 或其整倍数的片段,通过电泳可形成典型的"梯状带",而坏死细胞或凋亡后期的继发性坏死细胞 DNA 电泳后则成模糊的"涂片状"。

【应用】

快速和定性分析细胞凋亡现象,并可区分凋亡和坏死细胞。本实验是利用琼脂糖凝胶电泳分析小鼠胸腺淋巴细胞 DNA 在地塞米松诱导下细胞的凋亡现象。

【材料】

1. PBS
2. 细胞裂解液
3. 水饱和的酚、氯仿、异丙醇、冷无水乙醇
4. 6 mol/L NaI
5. 3 mol/L 醋酸钠
6. 10 mg/mL RNA 酶(无 DNA 酶活性)
7. TE 缓冲液(pH 8.0)
8. 50×TAE 电泳缓冲液
9. DNA ladder 分子量标准品
10. 6×凝胶加样缓冲液
11. 台式高速离心机、恒温水浴、全套琼脂糖凝胶电泳装置、凝胶电泳照相设备等

【方法】

待测细胞的制备:颈椎脱臼处死小鼠,无菌条件下取胸腺,去除小血管及结缔组织,

浸入含 5% 小牛血清的预冷 RPMI - 1640 培养液,16 号针头拉开胸腺,使细胞脱落, 250 μmt尼龙网过滤,1 000 r/min 离心 4 min,调节细胞浓度为 2×10^6 个/mL 待用。取上述 2×10^6 个/mL 浓度的胸腺细胞加入终浓度为 1×10^{-5} mol/L 的地塞米松,培养 5 h 即为凋 亡阳性细胞,对照组不加地塞米松。

1. 苯酚/氯仿提取 DNA 法:

(1) 将待测细胞用 PBS 洗一遍。

(2) 在 1.5 mL 微量离心管中,离心沉淀待测细胞,去除上清。

(3) 加入 50 μL 细胞裂解液,混匀,于 37℃水浴温育至混合物变得清亮。

(4) 在台式高速离心机中,以室温 12 000 r/min 离心 5 min,将上清转移至一洁净的 EP 管中。

(5) 以等体积的苯酚/氯仿(1:1)、苯酚/氯仿/异丙醇(25:24:1)和氯仿各抽提 一次。

(6) 在上清加入 1/10 体积 3 mol/L 醋酸钠和 2 倍体积冷乙醇,于-20℃沉淀过夜。

(7) 于 4℃ 12 000 r/min 离心 10 min,收集沉淀将沉淀溶于 20 μL TE 缓冲液,加入 1 μL RNA 酶,37℃温育 1 h。

(8) 加入 4 μL 样品缓冲液,混匀,立即加到含有 0.4 μg/mL 溴化乙锭的 1%~2% 的 琼脂糖凝胶的样品孔中,室温、恒流 75 mA,于 1×TAE 缓冲液中电泳 1~2 h,紫外灯下观察 实验结果并照相。

2. NaI 抽提 DNA 法:

(1) 同上(1)。

(2) 同上(2)。

(3) 加 dH$_2$O 200 μL,摇匀 20 s,加 6 mol/L NaI 200 μL,缓慢倒置摇匀 20 s。

(4) 加氯仿/异戊醇(24:1)400 μL,摇匀 20 s,12 000 r/min 离心 12 min。

(5) 吸取上层含 DNA 的水相 360 μL,置另一 EP 管中,加异丙醇 200 μL,摇匀 20 s, 室温放置 15 min,14 000 r/min 离心 12 min。

(6) 仔 细弃去上清,再加 37% 异 丙 醇 1 mL, 14 000 r/min离心 30 min。

(7) 小心弃去异丙醇,风干,加 25 μL TE 缓冲液溶 解 DNA。

(8) 同上(8)。

【结果】

加地塞米松培养的胸腺细胞 DNA 电泳后呈典型 的"阶梯状"条带,与标准分子量 DNA 参照物比较,为 多倍的 180~200 bp DNA 片段。未加加地塞米松培养 的胸腺细胞,DNA 无类似改变。细胞坏死对照的 DNA 电泳呈现弥漫的片状图谱(图 40-1)。

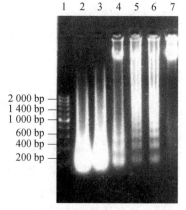

图 40 - 1　鼠胸腺凋亡细胞的 DNA
琼脂糖凝胶电泳分析

1. DNA marker;2~3. 细胞坏死对 照;4~6. 细胞凋亡;7. 正常细胞对照

【注意事项】

实验过程中,关键要防止 DNA 酶的作用和剧烈震荡造成 DNA 断裂。

【思考题】

为什么小鼠胸腺细胞用地塞米松诱导后易产生梯状 DNA 条带?

（章晓联）

Exp. 40   Thymocytes Apoptosis Assay by Agarose Gel Electrophoresis

【Principle】

Apoptosis is a physiological, programmed mode of cell death during body development. The distinct morphological changes of apoptosis are the internucleosomal DNA fragmentation by the stimulated restriction enzyme dependant on the changes of Ca^{2+}/Mg^{2+}. The distinct morphological feature of apoptotic cells is generation of $180-200$ bps unit or multiple oligonucleosomal fragments. The widespread methods for studying cell apoptosis include flow cytometry method, DNA agarose gel electrophoresis, isotope labelling of $3'$ end of DNA followed by electrophoresis and autoradiography, and in situ terminal deoxynucleotidyl transferase (TUNEL) method.

DNA agarose gel electrophoresis is a classical method of diagnosing biochemical changes of apoptosis. This method offers a sensitive, specific and rapid analysis. Apoptotic cells result in the degradation of the DNA into smaller $180-200$ bps units or its oligonucleosomal fragments and form a ladder pattern after electrophoresis of DNA. Apoptosis differs markedly from necrosis in which the changes associated with cell death arising from injury and forming a smear pattern after electrophoresis of DNA.

【Application】

To analyze cell apoptosis rapidly and qualitatively. This analysis method can separate apoptotic cells from necrotic cells. This experiment analyzes thymocyte apoptotic cells stimulated by dexamethasone qualitatively.

【Materials】

1. PBS
2. Cell lysates
3. Water saturated phenol, chloroform, isoamyl alcohol, cold absolute ethanol
4. 6 mol/L NaI
5. 3 mol/L NaAc
6. 10 mg/mL RNAase (No DNAase)
7. TE buffer (pH8.0)
8. 50×TAE electrophoresis buffer
9. DNA molecule ladder
10. 6×gel loading buffers

11. Bench high speed centrifuge, water bath, agarose gel electrophoresis apparatus, etc.

【Procedures】

Preparation of the sample cells: Kill the mouse by cervical vertebra dislocation. Take out the thymus under sterile manipulation. Get rid of the small vessels and the connective tissue. Put the thymus into pre-cold RPMI - 1640 (with 5% bovine serum). Rip it apart with $16^{\#}$ needle to make the cells fall off. Filter the mixture through 250 μm nylon mesh, Centrifuge the filtrate for 4 min at 1,000 r/min. Adjust the concentration of the cells to 2× 10^6/mL, add $1×10^{-5}$ mol/L dexamethasone and culture for 5 h to get apoptosis cells. The control group does not contain dexamethasone.

1. DNA extraction with phenol/chloroform method:

(1) Wash one time the cell with PBS.

(2) Centrifuge the cells in 1.5 mL micro-centrifuge tube, discard the supernatant.

(3) Add 50 μL cytolysis solutions, mix well, and keep the mixture at 37℃ water bath till it becomes clear.

(4) Centrifuge the mixture at 12,000 r/min for 5 min; transfer the supernatant to a clean micro-centrifuge tube.

(5) Extract DNA with equal volume of phenol/chloroform (1 : 1), phenol/chloroform/isopropanol (25 : 24 : 1) and chloroform respectively.

(6) Add one-tenth volume of 3 mol/L acetyl sodium and double volume of cold alcohol to the supernatant; store it at −20℃ for overnight.

(7) Centrifuge at 4℃ at 12,000 r/min for 10 min. Collect the precipitates and solve it in 20 μL TE buffer. Add 1 μL RNAase, keep it at 37℃ for 1 h.

(8) Add 4 μL sample buffer, mix well, then add the mixture quickly to sample well in 1%−2% agarose gel (with 0.4 μg/mL ethidium bromide in it). Electrophoresis in 1×TAE buffer at room temperature, 75 mA constant current for 1 − 2 h; Check the result under ultraviolet lamp and take a photo.

2. DNA extraction with NaI (Sodium Iodide) method:

(1) Same as above (1).

(2) Same as above (2).

(3) Add 200 μL dH$_2$O, shake 20 seconds, then add 200 μL NaI, slowly invert and shake 20 seconds.

(4) Add 400 μL chloroform/isopentanol (24 : 1), shake tubes 20 s then centrifuge them at 14,000 r/min for 12 min.

(5) Aspirate 360 μL of the upper water phase which has DNA in it and put it into another EP tube. Add pure isopropanol 200 μL, shake tubes 20 s. After 15 min at room temperature, centrifuge at 14,000 r/min for 12 min.

(6) Carefully discard the supernatant, then add 1 mL 37% isopropanol centrifuge at

14,000 r/min for 30 min.

(7) Discard the isopropanol carefully. Dry it in air then add 25 μL TE buffer to dissolve DNA.

(8) Same as above (8).

【Results】

The DNA from the thymocyte apoptotic cells stimulated by dexamethasone appeares "Ladder" pattern after electrophoresis (Lane 4 – 6 in Fig.40 – 1) and represents as multi 180 – 200 bp fragments. The DNA from the control cells without dexamethosone has no "Latter" pattern appeared (Lane 7 in Fig.40 – 1). While the DNA from necrosis cells appears a smear pattern after electrophoresis (Lane 2 – 3 in Fig.40 – 1).

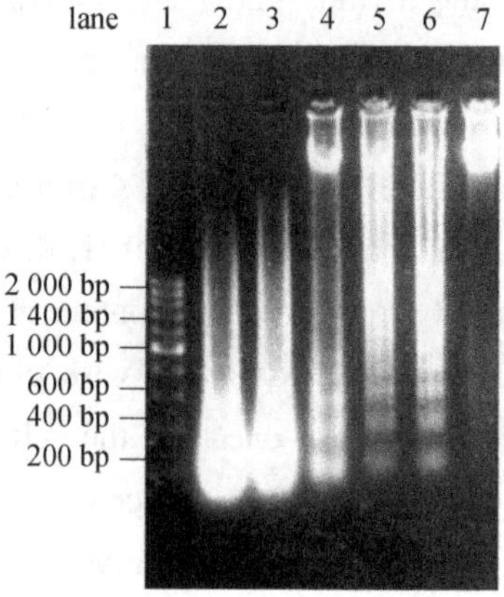

【Precautions】

Prevent contamination from DNAase and vigorously shake when extracting DNA.

【Question】

Why does thymocyte which is stimulated by dexamethasone easily form apoptotic cells and appear a ladder pattern when you run DNA agarose gel electrophoresis?

Fig. 40 – 1　DNA agarose gel electrophoresis analysis of mouse thymocyte apoptotic cells

1. DNA Molecular Marker; 2 – 3. Necrosis cells; 4 – 6. Apoptotic cells; 7. Control normal cells

(Zhang Xiaolian)

实验四十一　　流式细胞仪检测细胞凋亡
——Annexin V/PI 双染色法

【原理】

在正常细胞中,磷脂酰丝氨酸(PS)是一种带负电荷的磷脂,只分布在细胞膜脂质双层的内侧。在细胞凋亡早期,细胞膜中的 PS 由细胞膜脂质双层内侧翻向外侧。

Annexin V 是一种 Ca^{2+} 依赖的磷脂结合蛋白,与 PS 有高度亲和力,可通过细胞外侧暴露的 PS 与凋亡早期细胞的细胞膜结合。因此,Annexin V 可作为检测细胞早期凋亡的灵敏指标之一。将荧光素(EGFP、FITC)标记的 Annexin V 作为荧光探针,利用流式细胞仪检测细胞凋亡的发生。

碘化丙啶(PI)是一种核酸染料,不能透过完整的细胞膜,但在凋亡中晚期的细胞和坏死细胞中,PI 能够透过细胞膜与细胞核结合呈现红色。

因此,在细胞凋亡检测中联合使用 AnnexinV 与 PI,Annexin V 结合在细胞膜表面作为细胞凋亡的指示,PI 对凋亡中晚期的细胞和坏死细胞进行标记,可以将处于不同凋亡时期的细胞区分开来。

【应用】

流式细胞仪检测细胞凋亡可以用于:① 鉴定凋亡细胞形态;② 计数凋亡细胞数量;③ 细胞凋亡特异性定性和定量分析。

【材料】

1. Annexin V－FITC
2. 碘化丙啶(PI)
3. 0.25%胰酶消化液:胰蛋白酶 0.25 g,1×PBS 100 mL pH7.4
4. PBS 缓冲液(pH7.2~7.4):NaCl 137 mmol/L, KCl 2.7 mmol/L, Na_2HPO_4 10 mmol/L, KH_2PO_4 2 mmol/L
5. 连接缓冲液:HEPES/NaOH 10 mmol/L,pH7.4,NaCl 140 mmol/L,$CaCl_2$ 5 mmol/L
6. 标记液:将 Annexin V－FITC 和 PI 加入到连接缓冲液中,终浓度均为 1 μg/mL

【方法】

1. 细胞收集:贴壁细胞用不含 EDTA 的胰酶消化(注:胰酶消化时间不宜过长,否则容易引起假阳性),2 000 r/min 离心 5 min。
2. 用 PBS 洗涤细胞 2 次,2 000 r/min 离心 5 min,弃上清。
3. 用连接缓冲液洗涤一次,收集细胞数为(1~5)×10^6 个/mL, 2 000 r/min 离心 5 min,弃上清。

4. 用 100 μL 的标记溶液重悬细胞,室温下避光孵育 5~15 min。

5. 1 h 内进行流式细胞仪的观察和检测。

6. 流式细胞仪分析:流式细胞仪激发光波长用 488 nm,用一波长为 515 nm 的通带滤器检测 FITC 荧光,另一波长大于 560 nm 的滤器检测 PI(图 41 - 1)。

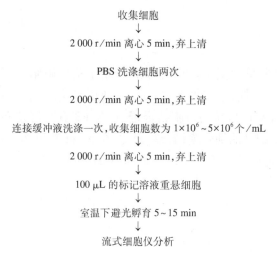

收集细胞
↓
2 000 r/min 离心 5 min,弃上清
↓
PBS 洗涤细胞两次
↓
2 000 r/min 离心 5 min,弃上清
↓
连接缓冲液洗涤一次,收集细胞数为 1×10⁶~5×10⁶ 个/mL
↓
2 000 r/min 离心 5 min,弃上清
↓
100 μL 的标记溶液重悬细胞
↓
室温下避光孵育 5~15 min
↓
流式细胞仪分析

图 41 - 1　流式细胞仪检测细胞凋亡流程示意图

【结果观察】

凋亡细胞对所有用于细胞活性鉴定的染料如 PI 有抗染性,坏死细胞则不能。细胞膜受损的细胞 DNA 可被 PI 染色产生红色荧光,而细胞膜保持完好的细胞则不会有红色荧光产生。因此,在细胞凋亡的早期 PI 不会染色,不会出现红色荧光信号。正常活细胞与此相似。在双变量流式细胞仪的散点图上,左下象限显示活细胞,为($FITC^-/PI^-$);右上象限是非活细胞,即坏死细胞,为($FITC^+/PI^+$);而右下象限为凋亡细胞,显现($FITC^+/PI^-$)。

【注意事项】

1. 未处理的对照细胞进行常规培养的过程中也有一小部分的细胞死亡发生。

2. Annexin V - FITC 和 PI 要避光保存及使用。

3. PI 有毒,操作时要戴手套。

4. 由于 Annexin-V 为 Ca^{2+} 依赖的磷脂结合蛋白,只有在 Ca^{2+} 存在的情况下与 PS 的亲和力才大,因而在消化贴壁细胞时,建议一般不采用含 EDTA 的消化液。

5. 必须设置阴性对照和补偿对照(分别单染)。

【思考题】

如何利用流式细胞仪检测 K562 细胞凋亡?

(邱文洪)

Exp. 41　Cell Apoptosis Test by Flow Cytometry — Annexin V/PI Dual Staining Method

【Principle】

In normal cells, phosphatidylserine (PS) is a negatively charged phospholipid that is only distributed inside the lipid bilayer of the cell membrane. In the early stage of apoptosis, PS in the cell membrane is turned to the outside from the inner side of the cell membrane lipid bilayer.

Annexin V is a Ca^{2+}-dependent phospholipid-binding protein that has a high affinity for PS. It can bind to the cell membrane of early apoptotic cells through PS exposed to the outside of the cell. Therefore, Annexin V can be used as one of the sensitive indicators for detecting early apoptosis of cells. Annexin V is labelled with fluorescein (EGFP, FITC), and the labelled Annexin V is used as a fluorescent probe, and apoptosis is detected by flow cytometry. Apoptosis can be detected by flow cytometry using Annexin V labeled with fluorescein (EGFP, FTTC), which is used as a flurescent probe.

Propidium iodide (PI) is a nucleic acid dye that does not penetrate intact cell membranes. However, in advanced apoptosis cells and necrotic cells, PI can communicate with the nucleus through the cell membrane and appears red.

Therefore, Annexin V and PI are combined in the detection of apoptosis. Annexin V binds to the surface of the cell membrane as an indicator of apoptosis. PI marks the cells in the middle and late stages of apoptosis, thus they can recognize cells at different stages of apoptosis.

【Application】

Detection of cell apoptosis by flow cytometry can be used to: ① identify apoptotic cells morphology; ② count the number of apoptotic cells; ③ analyze cell apoptosis qualitatively and quantitatively.

【Materials】

1. Annexin V－FITC
2. Propidium iodide(PI)
3. 0.25% trypsin digest liquid: trypsin 0.25 g, 1×PBS, 100 mL, pH 7.4
4. PBS (pH 7.2~7.4): NaCl 137 mmol/L, KCl 2.7 mmol/L, Na_2HPO_4 10 mmol/L, KH_2PO_4 2 mmol/L

5. Ligation buffer: HEPES/NaOH 10 mmol/L, pH7.4, NaCl 140 mmol/L, CaCl$_2$ 5 mmol/L

6. Labelling solution: add Annexin V – FITC and PI to the ligation buffer at a final concentration of 1 μg/mL

【Procedures】

1. Cell collection: adherent cells are digested with trypsin without EDTA (note: trypsin digestion time should not be too long, otherwise it is easy to cause false positive), cells are centrifuged at 2,000 r/min for 5 min.

2. Wash the cells twice with PBS, centrifuge cells at 2,000 r/min for 5 min, and discard the supernatant.

3. Wash once with binding buffer, collecting $(1-5) \times 10^6$/mL of cells, centrifuge cells at 2,000 r/min for 5 min, and discard the supernatant.

4. Resuspend the cells with 100 μL of labelling solution, incubating cells for 5 to 15 min at room temperature in the dark.

5. Observe and detect the cells by flow cytometry within 1 hour.

6. Flow cytometry analysis: using 488 nm wavelength of flow cytometer excitation light, FITC fluorescence is detected with a passband filter with a wavelength of 515 nm, and another filter with a wavelength greater than 560 nm is used to detect PI(Fig.41 – 1).

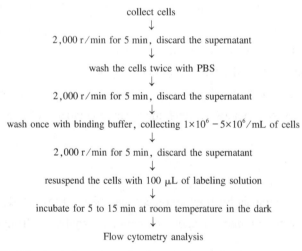

Fig.41 – 1   A flow chart of cell apoptosis test by flow cytometry

【Results】

Apoptotic cells are resistant to all dyes used for cell viability identification, such as PI, while necrotic cells are not. The DNA of cells with damaged cell membranes can be stained with PI to produce red fluorescence, while cells with intact cell membranes will not produce red fluorescence. Therefore, in the early stage of cell apoptosis, cells are not stained by PI with no red fluorescent signal. Normal living cells are similar. On the scatter plot of the bivariate flow cytometer, the lower left quadrant shows live cells as ($FITC^-/PI^-$); the upper right quadrant is non-viable cells, necrotic cells, ($FITC^+/PI^+$); and the lower right quadrant is apoptotic cells, visualized ($FITC^+/PI^-$).

【Precautions】

1. A small fraction of cell death is occurred during routine culture of untreated control cells.

2. Annexin V－FITC and PI should be protected from light.

3. PI is toxic and gloves should be worn during operation.

4. Because Annexin-V is a Ca^{2+}-dependent phospholipid-binding protein, it has a high affinity with PS only in the presence of Ca^{2+}. Therefore, during digesting adherent cells, it is recommended not to use EDTA-containing digestive buffer.

5. Negative controls and compensating controls (single dyeing, respectively) must be set.

【Question】

How can you use flow cytometry to identify cell apoptosis of K562 cells?

(Qiu Wenhong)

实验四十二　　流式细胞术检测小鼠 T 淋巴细胞亚群（CD4$^+$/CD8$^+$ T 细胞）

【原理】

流式细胞术（FCM）是一种检测液体流动相中通过激光束的细胞或微粒的技术。荧光标记抗体结合到混合细胞中表达相应抗原的细胞群,当细胞通过检测点时,荧光信号被捕捉,光信号如 FSC、SSC 荧光信号被转换为电信号（图 42 - 1）,因此,它被广泛用于细胞计数、形态学检测、生化信号检测和细胞悬液中个别细胞的标志物分析。

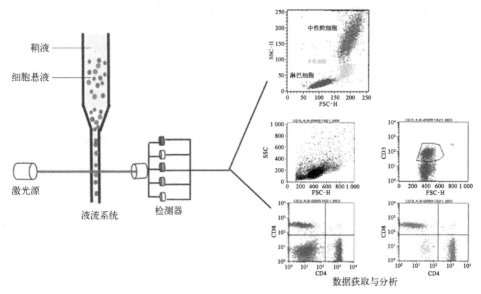

图 42 - 1　流式细胞仪结构和工作原理示意图

荧光包括细胞自发荧光（如核黄素、细胞色素等）,经荧光染料标记后的抗体分子结合到细胞表面或内部特异性分子（如 DNA、蛋白质等）形成的抗原-荧光抗体复合物等。常用荧光染料的激发波长见表 42 - 1。

表 42 - 1　常用于 FACS 的荧光染料及其波长特征

荧光染料	激发波长（nm）	发射波长（nm）
FITC	488	525（绿光）
PE	488	575（橙光）
PI	488	630（红光）
APC	633	660（红光）
PE-Cyanine 5.5	488	695（红光）

脾脏是外周免疫器官之一,含有大量巨噬细胞、T 淋巴细胞、B 淋巴细胞等免疫细胞,

是机体发挥细胞免疫和体液免疫应答的中心。CD3 阳性 T 细胞起源于骨髓多能干细胞,在胸腺中经过阳性选择和阴性选择后,分化为 CD4 或 CD8 单阳性 T 细胞后,进入外周免疫器官发挥 T 细胞介导的细胞免疫功能(图 42-2)。利用 CD3、CD4、CD8 等表面标志分子,通过不同荧光素标记的特异性抗体进行直接免疫荧光染色后,利用流式细胞仪检测,即可鉴定、分离和纯化相应的细胞亚群。

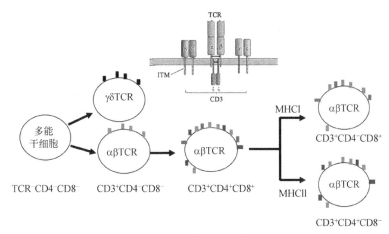

图 42-2　T 淋巴细胞的分化过程及其主要表面标记分子

　　本实验利用流式细胞仪测定结合于细胞表面的荧光标记抗体分子产生的荧光波长和强度,检测小鼠脾脏 T 淋巴细胞亚型 CD4 阳性或 CD8 阳性 T 细胞,进而掌握用 FCM 进行淋巴细胞亚型分类的方法。

【应用】

　　流式细胞术广泛应用于细胞或颗粒性物质的分类、分析及分选。例如,细胞的分类、分型、鉴定和表征;细胞周期、细胞凋亡。

【材料】

　　1. 0.01 mol/L PBS 溶液

　　2. 1% BSA 溶液

　　3. ACK 红细胞裂解液

　　4. 细胞培养液:RPMI-1640(GIBCO)+10%胎牛血清 FBS

　　5. 4%多聚甲醛

　　6. FACS 缓冲液

　　7. 抗体:FITC 标记的抗小鼠-CD4 抗体,PE 标记的抗小鼠-CD8a 抗体,APC 标记的抗小鼠-CD3e 抗体

【方法】

　　1. 小鼠脾脏细胞悬液制备:

　　(1) 颈椎脱臼法处死小鼠后,用浸有 75%乙醇的棉球擦拭小鼠腹部,然后用眼科剪依

次剪开小鼠腹部皮肤、筋膜、肌层。打开腹腔,可看到长 3~4 厘米呈长条状的深红色组织,即为脾脏。

（2）在 10 cm 培养皿中加入 5 mL 的 RPMI－1640 完全培养液,然后将分离得到的脾脏组织浸泡其中。取干净的注射器,用其针筒末端橡胶头对组织进行碾磨。

（3）用 5 mL 培养液清洗细胞筛,收集培养皿内细胞悬液,使其最终体积为 10 mL,转入 15 mL 离心管,1 000 r/min 离心 5 min,去上清;

（4）加入 1 mL 红细胞裂解液吹打混匀,室温裂解 3 min 以去除脾脏的红细胞;补加 9 mL 0.01 mol/L PBS 溶液,4℃ 1 000 r/min 离心 5 min,去上清。

（5）加入 1 mL FACS 缓冲液重悬细胞,细胞计数后,将细胞浓度调整为 $5 \times 10^6 \sim 10 \times 10^6$ 个/mL。

2. 荧光抗体染色分析:

（1）取上述稀释细胞悬液分别等量加入空白组、CD3、CD4 及 CD8 单染组,CD3+CD4 双染组、CD3+CD8 双染组或 CD3+CD4+CD8 三染组 EP 管中,确保每个 EP 管中细胞数量达到 $5 \times 10^5 \sim 10 \times 10^5$ 个/管。4℃ 1 000 r/min 离心 5 min,去上清。

（2）分别加 100 μL 稀释后的抗 CD3、CD4 或者 CD8 抗体溶液（5 μL 抗体+100 μL 1% BSA）,4℃避光孵育 30 min;然后加入 1 mL 1×PBS 溶液混匀,4℃ 1 000 r/min 离心 5 min,去上清。

（3）加入 500 μL 4%多聚甲醛,室温避光固定 15 min 后加入 500 μL 的 FACS 缓冲液,4℃ 1 000 r/min 离心 5 min,去上清。

（4）加入 800 μL FACS 缓冲液重悬细胞,在 24 h 内进行流式细胞仪检测。

3. 流式细胞仪检测和数据分析:

（1）打开 FACScan 电源,等待指示灯从 NOT READY 至 STANDBY。

（2）启动电脑连接 FACScan;打开桌面上的计数,选择合适的模板进行数据分析（参照说明书作正确设置）。将对照液体管置于流式细胞仪,按"RUN"按钮。

（3）将装有细胞的 FACS 测定管放置到机器吸管孔处。

（4）先预检测样品,然后进行实验检测。可根据细胞的浓度选择合适的测定速度。

（5）所有样品测定完后,用 FACS 清洁液、FACS 洗净液分别清洗仪器;最后用装有双蒸水的 FACS 管放置机器吸管。关闭机器。将废液槽中的废液倒掉,并清洗干净废液槽。

（6）使用 CELL QUEST 软件分析数据。

【结果】

用散点图显示数据结果,详细表述细胞的具体类型、比例及数量。

【注意事项】

1. 脾脏研磨过程要轻柔,否则会损伤脾脏细胞,研磨至细胞筛中不见整个脾脏细胞,只剩下一些不能磨碎的结缔组织为止。

2. 实验过程中保持低温以保证细胞活性。

3. 加入荧光标记抗体染色过程必须在 4℃避光进行。

4. 设置合适的对照组,其中每种荧光标记物都需设置单染色组,用于调节荧光间补偿。

5. 细胞与抗体相互作用后,一定要用缓冲液洗 2~3 次,以除去未结合的游离抗体。

6. 如果要同时检测两种以上的分子,一定要选择发射波长不同的荧光所标记的抗体。

7. 待测样品必须是单个细胞的悬液,如果有细胞团块,可用 70 μm 的细胞筛过滤后上机。

【思考题】

若同时检测细胞表面 2 个或更多参数(分子),如何设立对照? 如何分析数据?

(冯凌云)

Exp. 42 Mouse T Lymphocyte Subsets Analysis by Flow Cytometry (CD4$^+$/CD8$^+$ T Lymphocytes)

【Principle】

Flow cytometry (FCM) is a method allowing the analysis of various properties of cells or particles suspended in a fluid and flowing past a detector, where the stream is illuminated by a focused laser beam. Fluorescent dye-labelled antibodies which bind to specific cell associated antigen molecules in the mixed cell population are used for labelling. When the cells are illuminated by the laser through the detection point, scattered light from the fluorescent probe is detected, and part of the optical signal is converted into an electrical signal as FSC and SSC or the optical fluorescent wavelength shown in Fig.42 – 1. Thereby, it has been widely applied in cell counting, various morphologic detecting, biochemical signal dissection, and biomarker analysis of individual cell suspended in the flow.

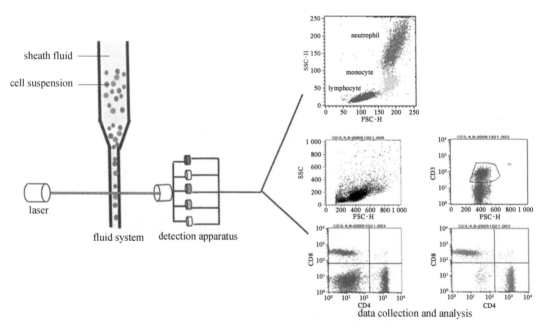

Fig.42 – 1   Schematic diagram of the basic structure and working principle of a flow cytometer

The fluorescence includes the spontaneous fluorescence of cells (such as riboflavin, cytochrome, etc.), and the fluorescent dyes which bind specifically onto the subcellular structure of the cell (such as DNA, protein, etc.) are labelled on antibodies which bind to the antigen molecules of the cell. The excitation and emission wavelength of the commonly used fluorescent dyes in FCM are shown in Tab. 42 − 1.

Tab. 42 − 1   Fluorescent dyes used in FACS and their wavelength characteristics

fluorescence dayes	excitation wavelengths(nm)	emission wavelengths(nm)
FITC	488	525(green)
PE	488	575(orange)
PI	488	630(red)
APC	633	660(red)
PE-Cyanine 5. 5	488	695(red)

Spleen is one of the predominantly peripheral immune organs, which contains a large number of immune cells, such as macrophages, T lymphocytes and B lymphocytes. It plays an important role during both cellular and humoral immune responses. CD3⁺ T cells originate from pluripotent stem cells in bone marrow and differentiate into CD4 or CD8 single positive mature T cells by positive selection and negative selection in the thymus, then enter the peripheral immune organs to involve in T cell-mediated immune response as shown in Fig.42 − 2. After direct immunofulorescence staining with CD3, CD4, CD8 and other surface marker molecules by specific antibody labelled with different luciferin, flow cytometry detection can be used to identity, isolate and purify the corresponding cell subsets.

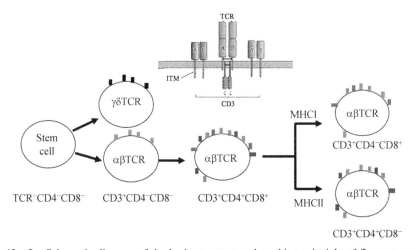

Fig.42 − 2   Schematic diagram of the basic structure and working principle of flow cytometer

In this experiment, the fluorescent-dye labelled antibodies are applied to detect the specific molecules on the surface of the mouse splenocytes and measured by flow cytometry. The CD4 positive Th cells or CD8 positive CTL cells of the splenic T lymphocyte subtypes in mice will be detected and classified by FCM.

【Application】

To analyze and classify cells or particles. Commonly used in DNA cell cycle analysis, apoptosis analysis and cell classification, etc.

【Materials】

1. 0.01 mol/L PBS (containing 0.1% sodium azide and 1% fetal bovine serum)

2. 1% BSA

3. ACK lysis buffer (0.15 mol/L NH_4Cl 0.4145 g, 10.0 mmol/L $KHCO_3$ 0.05 g, 0.1 mmol/L Na_2EDTA 1.86 mg. Add 30 mL H_2O and adjust pH to 7.2 - 7.4 with 1 mol/L HCl)

4. Culture medium: RPMI - 1640 (GIBCO) +10% fetal Bovine serum FBS

5. 4% paraformadehyde

6. FACS buffer

7. Antibodies: APC labeled anti-mouse CD3e, FITC-labeled anti-mouse CD4 and PE-labeled anti-mouse CD8a monoclonal antibodies

8. Flow cytometer

【Procedures】

1. Mouse splenocytes suspension preparation:

(1) After the mouse is sacrificed, remove the 3 - 4 cm long deep-red spleen from the abdomen of the mouse.

(2) Place the spleen into pre-moistened cell strainer in a 10 cm petri dish with 5 mL RPMI - 1640 containing 10% FBS media, and then grind the spleen with the rubber tip of the needle end of syringe.

(3) Clean the cell stainer with 5 mL media and collect the cell suspension in a 15 mL-centrifuge tube. Centrifuge cells at 1 000 r/min for 5 min and discard supernatant.

(4) Re-suspend the cell pellet in 1 mL of ACK lysis buffer and place at room temperature still for 3 min to remove RBCs from spleen. Then add 9 mL 1×PBS solution, centrifuge at 1 000 r/min for 5 min and discard supernatant.

(5) Re-suspend the cell pellet in 1 mL media, count cells using a cell counter, and adjust the cell concentration to $(0.5 - 1) \times 10^7$ cells/mL.

2. Preparation of the splenocyte samples for FACS assay:

(1) Add 1 mL FACS buffer into the suspension cells, and adjust cell concentration to $(5 - 10) \times 10^6$/mL.

(2) Separate $(5 - 10) \times 10^5$ cell suspensions into EP tubes of various groups, including the blank control, CD3, CD8 and CD4 single staining, $CD3^+CD4$ and $CD3^+CD8$ double staining, or $CD3^+CD4^+CD8$ triple staining. Centrifuge cells at 1 000 r/min, 4℃ for 5 min, then remove the supernatant.

(3) Add 100 μL of diluted anti-CD3, CD4 or CD8 antibody solution into each group and incubate tubes at 4℃ for 30 min in the dark; then add 1 mL of 0.01 mol/L PBS solution and mix well. Centrifuge cells at 1 000 r/min, 4℃ for 5 min. Discard supernatant.

(4) Fix the cells in 500 μL of 4% paraformaldehyde for 15 min at room temperature in the dark, and then add 500 μL of FACS buffer. Centrifuge cells at 1 000 r/min, 4℃ for 5 min, discard supernatant.

(5) Re-suspend the cells in 800 μL FACS buffer and perform flow cytometry analysis within 24 h.

3. Flow cytometry and data analysis:

(1) Turn on the FACScan power supply, and wait for the indicator light from NOT READY to STANDBY.

(2) Start the computer FACScan connection; open the count on the desktop and select the appropriate template for data analysis (refer to the manual for correct settings). Place the control tube on the flow cytometer and press the "RUN" button.

(3) Place the FACS tube containing the cells into the suction hole of the machine.

(4) Pre-test the sample and then conduct experimental testing. Select appropriate measurement speed to test all samples and collect the data as well.

(5) After all samples have been measured, clean the instrument with FACS cleaning solution and FACS cleaning solution. Finally, place the machine straw with a FACS tube with double distilled water before turn off the machine. Drain the waste from the waste tank and clean the waste tank.

(6) Analyze data with CELL QUEST software.

【Results】

Display data results with scatter plots. Describe the specific type, proportion and number of cells in detail.

【Precautions】

1. The spleen grinding process should be gentle; otherwise the spleen cells will be damaged. Grind until no spleen cells are visible in the cell strainer, leaving only connective tissue that can not be ground.

2. Keep the temperature low during the experiment to ensure cell viability.

3. The staining process with the addition of fluorescently labeled antibodies must be carried out at 4℃ in the dark.

4. The control groups should be set up, in which each fluorescent label is provided with a single dye tube for adjusting the fluorescence compensation.

5. After the antigen-antibody complex is formed, it is washed 2−3 times with a buffer for removing unbinding antibody.

6. If more than two molecules are detected at the same time, be sure to select antibodies labelled with different emission wavelengths of fluorescence.

7. The sample to be tested with FCM must be a suspension of a single cell. If there is a

cell mass, it can be filtered with a 70 μm cell strainer.

【Question】

If we need to analyze two or more parameters (surface molecules) on the cells at the same time, how to set up the control? How can we analyze the data?

(Feng Lingyun)

实验四十三　流式细胞术检测 CD4$^+$ T 细胞上 CXCR4 的表达

【原理】

流式细胞术(FCM)是一种对液流中悬浮的细胞或颗粒的性质进行多参数分析的方法。细胞流通过检测点时被聚焦的激光束照射。细胞通常被结合特异性表面分子的荧光探针所标记。

当细胞流通过检测点被激光束照射时,检测到荧光探针发出的散射光,部分光信号被转换成电信号,这样可以检测细胞流中悬浮的单个细胞的多种表型、生化及分子特性。细胞通过激光束时发出散射光,可以检测单个细胞的大小及颗粒性质。

FCM 能够通过测定可见光和荧光的发射对单个活(或死)细胞进行快速、定量、多参数分析。

本实验的基本原理在于检测结合特异细胞表面分子的荧光标记抗体产生的荧光强度,以检测 CD4$^+$ T 细胞表面的 CXCR4 的表达为例,了解 FCM 检测样本的方法。

【应用】

FCM 可用于细胞或颗粒的分析及分类,常用于 DNA 细胞周期分析、细胞凋亡分析、绿色荧光蛋白细胞分类、胞内铁蛋白测定、细胞间连接物测定和免疫表型分析等。

【材料】

1. 染液：PBS(含 0.1%叠氮化钠和 1%的胎牛血清)
2. 荧光标记抗体：PE 标记抗人 CXCR4 单抗和 PE 标记的同种型匹配单抗
3. 5 mL 聚苯乙烯管
4. 固定液：1%多聚甲醛(PBS 配)
5. 离心机
6. 可调微量移液器
7. 涡旋混匀器
8. 带盖冰桶
9. 流式细胞仪(FACScan)

【方法】

1. 使用 CD4 - Dynabeas M - 450 将人外周血单个核细胞中的 CD4$^+$T 细胞纯化。
2. 取 100~200 μL 经 PBS 重悬的 CD4$^+$T 细胞悬液(1×10^{6}个/mL)置于每一试管底部。
3. 分别将 5 μg/mL 的 PE -抗 CXCR4 单抗和 PE -同种型单抗加入上述试管内。
4. 轻轻摇匀,置于冰桶中,避光孵育 20~30 min。

5. PBS 洗涤细胞 2 次,涡旋混匀,2 000 r/min 离心 5 min。

6. 每管加 500 μL PBS,涡旋混匀,用于分析。细胞可储存于 1% 多聚甲醛,置 2~8℃ 保存 1 周以内,尽快进行分析。

7. 流式细胞仪分析:

(1) 打开 FACScan 电源,等待指示灯从"NOT READY"至"STANDBY"。重新启动电脑 FACScan 连接。

(2) 打开桌面上的计数,选择合适的模板进行数据分析(参照说明书作正确设置)。

(3) 将对照液体管置于流式细胞仪,按"RUN"按钮,一般来说,实验者可从每一样品获得 5 000 至 15 000 个细胞。

(4) 使用 CELL QUEST 软件分析数据。

【结果】

用单参数直方图显示数据结果(图 43-1)。横坐标显示荧光密度以对数增长,纵坐标表示细胞数。与 PE 标记的抗 CXCR4 单抗呈阳性反应的细胞如图中 2 所示;PE 标记的同种型单抗作为阴性对照的结果如图中 1 所示。横坐标上的虚线明确了特异性阴性反应细胞的范围(最低敏感限度)。

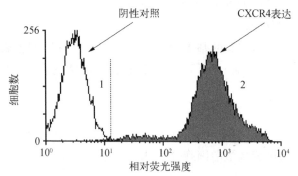

图 43-1   流式细胞术检测 CD4⁺T 细胞上 CXCR4 的表达

荧光指数(FI)= 检测样品的平均荧光强度/阴性对照的平均荧光强度。

FI>1 表明细胞上待测分子表达高。FI 值越大,表明待测分子的表达越多。

【注意事项】

1. 待测样品必须是单个细胞的悬液。

2. 连接的抗体剂量通常为 $1×10^6$ 个细胞不超过 1 μg。由于应用范围的不同,每位操作者必须确定每种检测样品的适当稀释度。

3. 染色过程必须在 4℃ 进行,避光。合适的对照才能得到正确的结果。若同时用 2 种或更多的抗体标记细胞,每种荧光标记物都需设对照。

4. 细胞应 4℃ 保存。若不立即检测,应将细胞固定于 1% 多聚甲醛中。

【思考题】

1. 上述方法是一种直接染色法,你知道如何通过间接染色法进行流式细胞仪分析吗?

2. 试检测甲醛固定细胞前后荧光强度是否存在差异,并分析其原因。

(李　群)

Exp. 43 Flow Cytometry Assay for CXCR4 Expression on CD4$^+$ T Cell

【Principle】

Flow cytometry is a method allowing the analysis of various properties of cells or particles suspended in a fluid, which flows past a detector point, where the stream is illuminated by a focused laser beam. The cells are usually labelled with fluorescent probes which bind to specific cell associated molecules.

As the cells flow past the detector point and the fluoresce probes are illuminated; the emitted light is detected and converted into electronic signals proportional to the amount of light collected. In this way, measurements of various phenotypic, biochemical and molecular characteristics of individual cells (or particles) suspended in a fluid stream are possible. Data regarding the relative size and granularity of a cell are also obtained due to the scattered light as the cell passes through the laser beam.

Flow cytometry can provide rapid, quantitative, multiparameter analyses on single living (or dead) cells based on the measurement of visible and fluorescent light emission.

This basic protocol focuses on measurement of fluorescence intensity produced by fluorescent-labled antibodies and ligands that bind specific cell-associated molecules. Here we take analysis of CXCR4 expression on CD4$^+$ T cells using flow cytometer as an example to show how to detect the sample using flow cytometry.

【Application】

Applications of flow cytometry are broadly divided into the analysis and sorting of cells or particles. Frequent applications include DNA cell cycle analysis, apoptosis analysis, green fluorescent protein cell sorting, measurement of intracellular ions, measurement of intercellular conjugates and immunophenotyping, etc.

【Materials】

1. Staining solution: PBS (containing 0.1% Sodium Azide and 1% FCS)
2. Fluorescent-labelled antibodies: PE conjugated anti-human CXCR4 mAb and PE conjugated isotype-matched mAb
3. Polystyrene tube of 5 mL
4. Fixation solution: 1% paraformaldehyde in PBS
5. Centrifuge
6. Precision adjustable micropipette

7. Vortex mixer

8. Ice bucket with cover

9. Flow cytometer (FACScan)

【Procedures】

1. Purify CD4$^+$ T cells from PBMC using CD4 - Dynabeads M450 (Dynal, Oslo, Norway).

2. Add 100 - 200 μL of CD4$^+$ T cell suspension (1×10^6 cells /mL) in PBS to the bottom of each tube.

3. Add the PE-anti-CXCR4 mAb with 5 μg /mL and PE-isotype-matched mAb with 5 μg/mL to each tube containing cell suspension, respectively.

4. Shake cells gently and incubate in the dark on the ice for 20 - 30 minutes.

5. Wash cells by adding excessive PBS, vortex and centrifuge cells 5 min at 2,000 r / min. Remove supernatant, resuspend cells in PBS, and repeat the wash once again.

6. Add 500 μL PBS to each tube and vortex for analysis. Cells can be stored in 1% paraformaldehyde at 2 - 8℃ for up to 1 week prior to analysis.

7. Flow cytometry analysis：

(1) Turn on the FACScan power and wait until the indicator light changes from NOT READY to STANDBY. Restart the computer to connect with the FACScan.

(2) Open your account on the desktop and use the appropriate template for acquiring data (see reference for making correct setting).

(3) Turn fluid control valve to RUN and place sample tube on FACScan. Typically, investigators acquire 5,000 to 15,000 cells per sample.

(4) Analyze data with CELLQuest Software.

【Results】

The data is shown by single parameter fluorescence histograms(Fig.43 - 1). Increasing fluorescence intensity is plotted on the *X* axis in log fluorescence unites versus cell number on the *Y* axis. Cells are reacted with positive PE-anti-CXCR4 mAb (2), or with negative control PE-isotype-matched mAb (1). The dashed line drawn at the *X* axis value defines the region of specifically negative cells (the lower limit of interest).

Fluorescence index (FI) = the mean fluorescence intensity of the experiment sample divided by the

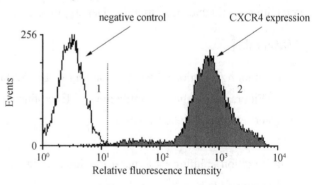

Fig.43 - 1   Flow cytometry analysis for expression of CXCR4 on CD4$^+$ T cells

mean fluorescence intensity of the negative control.

FI>1 means that the molecule interested is up-regulated on the cells. The bigger FI is, the higher up regulated the interested molecule is.

【Precautions】

1. The sample must be in monodisperse (single cell) suspension.

2. The dose of antibody conjugate is usually used below 1 μg /million cells. Each investigator must determine dilutions appropriate for individual use.

3. The staining procedure is carried out at 4℃ and dark. Appropriate controls are needed to get correct results. If you're planning to label cells with 2 or more antibodies simultaneously, you need a negative control for each fluorochrome conjugate.

4. Keep the cells on ice, covered, until your scheduled time on the flow cytometer. If you can not detect the samples right now, please fix the cells with 1% paraformaldehyde.

【Questions】

1. This procedure is a kind of direct staining method. Can you introduce an indirect staining way to prepare the sample for flow cytometry analysis?

2. Try to detect and analyze the difference in fluorescence intensity before and after formaldehyde-fixed cells.

(Li Qun)

实验四十四　流式细胞仪检测巨噬细胞胞内细胞因子

【原理】

巨噬细胞来源于血液循环中的单核细胞,这些单核细胞由骨髓产生,巨噬细胞特异性的表面标记分子为 F4/80。单核细胞在血液中仅停留 8 h 左右,然后穿过血管内皮,迁移到不同的组织并分化为长寿命的组织特异性的巨噬细胞。机体在外源因素的感染刺激下,巨噬细胞可以极化为两种不同的类型,即 M1 型或 M2 型。M1 型巨噬细胞是经典活化的巨噬细胞,M2 型巨噬细胞则是选择性活化的巨噬细胞。这两种巨噬细胞能分泌不同的细胞因子,行使不同的功能。在体外条件下,LPS 和 INF－γ 能刺激巨噬细胞向 M1 型极化,并释放 IL－1,IL－12 和 TNF－α 等细胞因子,发挥促炎作用。而 M2 型巨噬细胞则由 IL-4 和 IL－13 刺激形成,其能分泌大量 IL－10,但 IL－12 的表达水平降低,主要参与组织修复。因此,巨噬细胞分泌的细胞因子的变化,能体现细胞的状态及功能变化。细胞因子的检测有多种方法,本实验使用流式细胞仪检测 M1 型巨噬细胞内特异性胞内因子IL－12 的表达。

对于胞内细胞因子的检测,为了阻止细胞因子分泌到细胞外,增加其在胞内的含量,需要在培养基中加入转运抑制剂。收集到的细胞需经过固定、破膜等步骤,进行胞内细胞因子染色(图 44－1)。

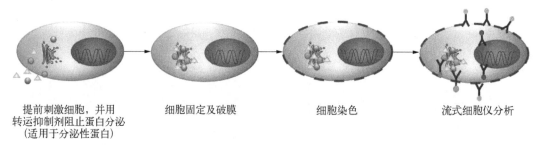

提前刺激细胞,并用　　　　细胞固定及破膜　　　　细胞染色　　　　流式细胞仪分析
转运抑制剂阻止蛋白分泌
（适用于分泌性蛋白）

图 44－1　胞内因子染色原理(图片来源于 BD 公司网站)

【应用】

流式细胞仪检测巨噬细胞内细胞因子。

【材料】

1. C57BL/6 小鼠
2. 转运抑制剂 Brefeldin A
3. 固定剂(4%多聚甲醛)
4. 破膜剂

5. 0.5 mmol/L EDTA·4Na

6. RPMI-1640 培养液(含 10%胎牛血清)

7. PBS

8. LPS 和小鼠来源的 IFN-γ 细胞因子

9. APC-F4/80、PE-IL-12 单克隆抗体及该抗体的同型对照抗体

10. 离心管、血细胞计数板、流式管、试管、吸管、滤网、水浴箱、离心机、流式细胞仪等

【方法】

1. 骨髓来源巨噬细胞(BMDM)的获取(参考实验十一)。

2. 将分离诱导得到的 BMDM 计数后铺六孔板,每孔 $1.5×10^6$ 个细胞,37℃培养 6 h。

3. 待 BMDM 细胞贴壁后,加入 100 ng/mL LPS 和 20 ng/mL 鼠源 IFN-γ 细胞因子刺激 48 h,以不刺激 BMDM 作为对照。

4. 在刺激结束前 6 h 加入 Brefeldin A。

5. 刺激时间到后,去除培养液,用 PBS 洗 1 遍。每孔加入 1 mL 0.5 mmol/L EDTA·4Na, 37℃消化 20 min。

6. 1 000 r/min 离心 5 min 后弃上清,100 μL PBS 重悬细胞。

进行流式检测前进行细胞染色分组:① 未刺激 BMDM 未染组;② 未刺激 BMDM, APC-F4/80 染色;③ 未刺激 BMDM, APC-F4/80+PE-isotype 染色;④ 未刺激 BMDM, APC-F4/80+PE-IL-12 染色;⑤ 刺激 BMDM, APC-F4/80+PE-isotype 染色;⑥ 刺激 BMDM, APC-F4/80+PE-IL-12 染色。

7. 根据分组情况,① 组 4℃放置不做处理,待上机,②~⑥组分别进行巨噬细胞表面标记 F4/80 染色,每组分别加入 5 μL APC-F4/80,避光 4℃染色 30 min。

8. 染色结束后,每组加入 2 mL 预冷 PBS,1 000 r/min 离心 5 min,每组加入 300 μL 固定剂,室温避光固定 15 min。

9. 固定时间结束后,加入 2 mL 预冷 PBS,1 000 r/min 离心 5 min,弃去液体。③~⑥组再加入 2 mL 含有破膜剂的 PBS 洗 2 遍。

10. PBS 重悬细胞,③~⑥分别加入 5 μL PE 标记的同型对照及 IL-12 流式抗体,避光 4℃染色 30 min。

11. 染色完成后,加入预冷 PBS 洗涤细胞后,1 000 r/min 离心 5 min,弃去 PBS。

12. 用 200~400 μL PBS 重悬细胞,①~⑥组细胞均经 300 目滤网过滤后,用流式细胞仪检测。

【结果】

流式细胞仪检测,根据未染、单染以及同型对照染色的细胞调整流式细胞仪电压及荧光通道的电压。选定 APC-F4/80 标记的阳性 BMDM 细胞,比较刺激或是未刺激情况下巨噬细胞胞内细胞因子 IL-12 的表达情况。

【注意事项】

1. 需提前向培养液中加入转运抑制剂,并培养一段时间。
2. 实验需设置各种对照,包括未染细胞对照及同型对照以降低非特异性染色。
3. 流式细胞仪上机前需将细胞过滤,分散为单细胞悬液。

【思考题】

1. 如果用流式细胞仪检测 M2 型巨噬细胞的细胞因子表达情况,应选用哪一种细胞因子?
2. 在免疫抑制环境中,哪一种类型的巨噬细胞占多数?

(赵颖岚　向　田)

Exp. 44　Flow Cytometer Analysis for Intracellular Cytokine of Macrophage

【Principle】

Macrophages are raised from circulating monocytes which originate from bone marrow. The specific surface marker molecule of macrophages is F4 /80. Monocytes remain in the blood for only about eight hours, then pass through the endothelium, migrate to different tissues and differentiate into long-lived tissue-specific macrophages. Macrophages are polarized into two subset (M1 and M2) by the stimuli present in the extracellular matrix. *In vitro*, M1 macrophage is stimulated by LPS and INF-γ, it is also called classical activated macrophage; while M2 macrophage which is stimulated by IL-4 and IL − 13, is called alternative activated macrophage. Once be polarized to M1 or M2, they will produce different cytokines and conduct different function. M1 macrophage mainly produces IL − 1, IL − 12 and TNF − α, which function as proinflammation activity. In contrast, activation of M2 macrophage leads to secretion of high amounts of IL − 10 and low levels of IL − 12 which promote tissue repair. Therefore, cytokines secreted by macrophages can be used to indicate its function. In this experiment, flow cytometer is used to measure the expression level of a specific macrophage intracellular cytokine − IL − 12.

For intracellular cytokine analysis, transport inhibitors should be added into culture medium to prevent cytokine secretion into the medium. After that, cells must be fixed and subjected to permeabilization condition to allow the entry of antibody. Then, intracellular cytokine can be stained by fluorescent labelled cytokine-specific antibody and analyzed by flow cytometer(Fig.44 − 1).

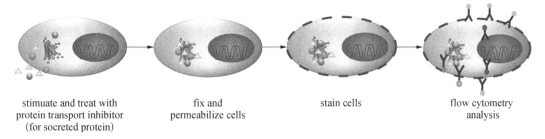

stimuate and treat with protein transport inhibitor (for socreted protein)　　fix and permeabilize cells　　stain cells　　flow cytometry analysis

Fig.44 − 1　Basic principle of intracellular cytokine staining (from BD Science company website)

【Application】

Using flow cytometer to detect macrophage intracellular cytokine (IL − 12).

【Materials】

1. C57BL/6 mice
2. Brefeldin A
3. Fixation buffer (4% paraformaldehyde)
4. Permeabilization wash buffer
5. 0.5 mmol/L EDTA · 4Na
6. RPMI－1640 supplementary with 10% FBS
7. PBS
8. LPS and Mouse-derived IFN-γ
9. APC－F4/80, PE－IL－12 monoclonal antibodies and isotype control antibodies
10. Centrifuge tube, hemocytometer, sample tubes of flow cytometer, test tube, pipette, cell strainer water bath, centrifuge, flow cytometer, etc.

【Procedures】

1. Harvest bone marrow derived macrophage (BMDM) as experiment 11.

2. Count cells with hemocytometer, then seed BMDM into 6-well plate (1.5×10^6/well) and cultured BMDM at 37℃ for 6 hours.

3. Add 100 ng/ml LPS and 20 ng/mL IFN-γ to stimulate polarization of BMDM for 48 hours, set untreated cells as control.

4. Add Brefeldin A 6 h at the end of the stimulation.

5. After stimulation, the medium is removed and washed 1 time with PBS. Digest each well with 1 mL 0.5 mmol/L EDTA · 4Na and incubate at 37℃ for 20 minutes.

6. Centrifuge at 1 000 r/min for 5 minutes, discard supernatant, resuspend cell with PBS (10^6 cells/100 μL PBS).

7. Cells are divided into several groups as below: ① BMDM without stimulation; ② BMDM without stimulation: stained by APC－F4/80; ③ BMDM without stimulation: stained by APC－F4/80 and PE-isotype; ④ BMDM without stimulation: stained by APC－F4/80 and PE－IL－12; ⑤ stimulated BMDM: stained by APC－F4/80 and PE-isotype; ⑥ stimulated BMDM: stained by APC－F4/80 and PE－IL－12.

8. Leave group① at 4℃, other groups are stained with 5 μL macrophage surface marker APC－F4/80 and then cells are stained at 4℃ in dark for 30 min.

9. Wash cells with 2 mL pre-cold PBS, centrifuge cells at 1 000 r/min for 5 minutes, decant liquid. Fix cells in 300 μL fixation buffer in the dark for 15 minutes at room temperature.

10. Wash cells with 2 mL pre-cold PBS, centrifuge cells at 1 000 r/min for 5 minutes, discard fixation buffer. Wash cells with 2 mL permeabilization wash buffer containing PBS twice.

11. Resuspend cell with PBS, add 5 μL PE-isotype and PE – IL – 12 antibody, cells are stained at 4℃ for 30 minutes in dark (group③–⑥).

12. Wash cells with 2 mL pre-cold PBS, centrifuge cells at 1,000 r/min for 5 minutes, discard liquid.

13. Resuspend the cells in 200 – 400 μL PBS buffer and transfer to test tube through filter membrane for flow cytometric analysis.

【Results】

Set flow cytometry according to unstained, single stained and isotype stained cells, adjust voltage that most suitable forward and and side scatter. Both APC – F4/80 and PE – IL – 12 positive BMPM cells are selected and analyzed under stimulated or unstimulated condition.

【Precautions】

1. Transport inhibitors should be added into culture medium and incubate cells as indicating time (each cytokine is different).

2. Do not forget to set an isotype negative control to reduce non-specific binding.

3. Filter the cells to get single cell suspension before flow cytometric analysis.

【Questions】

1. Which type of cytokine we can use to identify M2 macrophage population?

2. In immune repressive enviroment, which type of macrophage is in majority?

(Zhao Yinglan   Xiang Tian)

Chapter Eight

糖免疫技术
Glycoimmunology Technique

实验四十五　　IgG 糖链检测

【原理】

免疫球蛋白 G（IgG）含有 $N-$ 的糖链（通常位于 IgG 的 Fc 的 Asn_{297} 位）。依据该 $N-$ 糖链末端 Gal 糖基组成不同,有三种糖型 IgG:IgG G_0 糖型（两条糖链末端均缺 Gal,暴露出次末端的 GlcNAc 糖基）,IgG G_1 糖型（两条糖链末端缺失一个 Gal）,IgG G_2 糖型（两条糖链的末端都具有 Gal）(图 45-1)。根据凝集素能与特定的末端寡糖特异结合的原理,即可采用仅能与末端 GlcNAc 特异反应的 Griffonia simplicifolia（GS II）,也可采用能与末端 Manβ1-2GlcNAc 特异反应的 Psathyrella Velutina Lectin（PVL）,识别 $N-$ 糖链末端暴露出 GlcNAc 的 G_0 糖型。类风湿关节炎（RA）患者血清中 IgG G_0 糖型比例明显高于健康人的,且增高的程度与 RA 患者的病理症状密切相关。根据凝集素能与特定的末端寡糖特异结合的原理,可通过 ELISA 方法检测 RA 患者血清 IgG G_0 糖型。

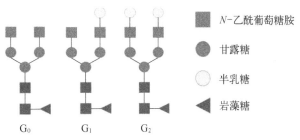

图 45-1　IgG G_0、IgG G_1 和 IgG G_2 的示意图

【应用】

IgG 中 G_0 糖型的增加对于 RA 的早期诊断具有重要意义。G_0 糖型的增高先于 RA 临床症状出现,并且 G_0 糖型增高的程度与 RA 患者炎症加重、RA 病理和病情复发密切相关,在临床的预后判断上具有一定的意义。

【材料】

1. 毡毛小脆柄菇凝集素（PVL）
2. 牛血清白蛋白（BSA）
3. HRP 标记抗人 IgG 抗体
4. 邻苯二胺（OPD）
5. 分离血清 IgG 样本
6. PBST（含 0.05% 吐温-20 的 PBS）
7. OPD 缓冲液:pH4.0,$Na_2HPO_3 \cdot 12H_2O$ 1.43 g,柠檬酸 0.63 g,加三蒸水至 100 mL
8. 2 mol/L H_2SO_4

【方法】

1. 以 PBS 稀释 PVL 至 5 mg/L,每孔加 PVL 稀释液 75 μL 包被酶标板（条）,4℃

过夜。

 2. PBST 洗 4 次。

 3. 加入 1% BSA 200 μL，在 37℃恒温箱中孵育 30 min。

 4. 直接加入 75 μL 血清 IgG 样本，在 37℃恒温箱中孵育 2 h。

 5. PBST 洗 4 次。

 6. 加入 75 μL HRP 标记的抗人 IgG 抗体，在 37℃恒温箱中孵育 1 h。

 7. PBST 洗 5 次。

 8. 加入 75 μL OPD－H_2O_2，在 37℃恒温箱中孵育 10 min。

 9. 2 mol/L H_2SO_4 终止反应。

 10. 在酶标仪上 490 nm 读取 OD 值。

【结果】

肉眼观察，待测标本明显高于健康对照而呈黄色则可判断阳性。也可以测定光密度（OD_{490}），判断待测样品是否为阳性。

【注意事项】

凝集素包被酶标板，不是必须在 4℃过夜的条件下进行，亦可在 37℃时，反应 90 min 即可，以缩短反应时间。

【思考题】

除了利用凝集素 ELISA 方法检测 G_0 糖型以外，还有什么比较常见的检测方法？

（刘　鹏　章晓联）

Exp. 45   Assay of IgG Sugar Chain

〖Principle〗

Immunoglobulin G (IgG) contains N-linked sugar chains (usually at Asn_{297} position of IgG Fc fragment). According to the different composition of N-glycan terminal galactose glycosyl, three glycoforms of G_0, G_1 and G_2 glycoforms are shown as in Fig.45 − 1.

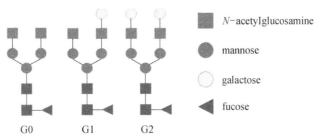

Fig.45 − 1   Schematic diagram of three glycoforms
of IgG G_0, G_1 and G_2

Different lectins bind to different terminal sugars. For example, Griffonia simplicifolia (GSII) can specifically react with the terminal N-acetyglucosamin (GlcNAc) (IgG G_0 glycoform), and Psathyrella Velutina Lectin (PVL) can also specifically react with the terminal $Man\beta1 - 2GlcNAc$ (IgG G_0 glycoform). So IgG G_0 glycoform with terminal GlcNAc at the end of the N-glycan chain can be identified with GSII and PVL. Serum samples of rheumatoid arthritis (RA) patients contain higher percentage of IgG G_0 glycoforms comparing with those of the healthy donors. Based on the characteristics of PVL or GSII which can specifically bind to specific terminal GlcNAc, the IgG G_0 glycoform of RA patients can be detected by these specific lectins with ELISA.

〖Application〗

The increasing ratio of glycoform G_0 in IgG is important for the early diagnosis of RA. The increasing of glycoform G_0 appears before the clinical symptoms of RA, and the increased degree of G_0 glycoform is closely related to the inflammation in RA patients, as well as the pathological characteristics and recurrence of RA.

〖Materials〗

1. Psathyrella velutina lectin (PVL)
2. Bovine serum albumin(BSA)
3. HRP-labeled anti-human IgG antibody

4. O-phenylenediamine(OPD)

5. Isolated serum IgG samples

6. PBST (PBS containing 0.05% Tween-20)

7. OPD buffer: pH 4.0, $Na_2HPO_3 \cdot 12H_2O$ 1.43 g, citric acid 0.63 g, add three steamed water to 100 mL

8. 2 mol/L H_2SO_4

【Procedures】

1. Dilute PVL to 5 mg/L in PBS, add 75 μL of the PVL dilution solution into each well, and then coat the plate (strip) at 4℃ overnight.

2. Wash the plate with PBST 4 times.

3. Add 200 μL of 1% BSA and incubate plate in a 37℃ incubator for 30 min.

4. Add 75 μL of serum IgG samples directly and incubate plate in a 37℃ incubator for 2 h.

5. Wash 4 times with PBST.

6. Add 75 μL of HRP-labelled anti-human IgG antibody and incubate plate in a 37℃ incubator for 1 h.

7. Wash with PBST 5 times.

8. Add 75 μL of OPD − H_2O_2 and incubate in a 37℃ incubator for 10 min.

9. Terminate the reaction by adding 2 mol/L H_2SO_4.

10. Read the OD value at 490 nm with a microplate reader.

【Results】

Yellow color shown in the specimen is presented as positive when its color is significantly higher than those of healthy controls. The optical density (OD_{490}) can also be measure for evaluating positive results.

【Precautions】

The lectin coated on the ELISA plate is carried out at 4℃ overnight, or at 37℃ for 90 min.

【Question】

Beside ELISA, are there any other methods used to detect the G_0 glycoform of IgG?

(Liu Peng　Zhang Xiaolian)

实验四十六　　免疫球蛋白 A1 糖链的检测

【原理】

免疫球蛋白 A(IgA)有 IgA1 和 IgA2 两种亚型,以 IgA1 亚型为主。IgA1 是高度糖基化的,在铰链区有 4~5 个 O-糖化位点,形成 O-糖链簇。其 O-糖链具有如下结构:NeuNAc-Gal-GalNAc-O-Ser(Thr),而缺失末端 Gal、暴露出次末端的 GalNAc 的异常 O-糖链,与 IgA 肾病的病理症状密切相关。

根据凝集素能与特定的末端寡糖特异结合的原理,采用能特异与末端 GalNAc 反应的 Helix aspersa(HAA),识别该 O-糖链末端暴露出 GalNAc 的异常 IgA1 糖型,通过 ELISA 夹心法对其进行检测。此外,也可应用生物素—凝集素反应体系,通过 Western-blotting 方法进行检测。

【应用】

在 IgA 肾病患者体内,由于异常血清 IgA1 先于临床症状出现,并直接反映肾脏损伤程度,与治疗效果及预后判断均密切相关,因此检测异常血清 IgA1 被认为是理想的诊断 IgA 肾病的方法之一。

【材料】

1. 螺旋蜗牛(HAA)
2. 牛血清白蛋白(BSA)
3. 碱性磷酸酶(AP)标记的抗人 IgA 抗体
4. 对硝基苯磷酸盐法(PNPP)
5. PBS
6. PBST:在 PBS 中加入吐温-20 至浓度为 0.05%
7. 碱性磷酸酶(AP)缓冲液(pH9.5),NaCl 5.8 g,$MgCl_2$ 1.0 g,Tris 12.1 g,加三蒸水定容至 1 000 mL
8. TBS:Tris 12.114 g,NaCl 9.00 g,加三蒸水定容至 1 000 mL,HCl 调 pH 为 8.0 左右,4℃保存
9. 1 mo/L NaOH
10. 酶标仪
11. 酶标板(条)
12. 电子天平
13. 恒温水浴箱

【方法】

1. ELISA 方法检测 IgA1 异常糖型:

(1) 以 TBS 稀释 HAA 至 5 mg/L,每孔加 HAA 稀释液 75 μL 包被酶标板(条),4℃

过夜。

(2) PBST 洗 4 次。

(3) 加入 200 μL 1% BSA,在 37℃水浴箱中保温 30 min。

(4) 直接加入 75 μL 血清,在 37℃水浴箱中保温 2 h。

(5) PBST 洗 4 次。

(6) 加入 75 μL AP 标记的抗人 IgA 抗体,在 37℃水浴箱中保温 1 h。

(7) PBST 洗 5 次。

(8) 加入 75 μL PNPP,在 37℃水浴箱中保温 30 min。

(9) 加 50 μL 1 mol/L NaOH 终止反应。

(10) 在酶标仪上 405 nm 读取 OD 值。

2. Western blotting 方法检测 IgA1 异常糖链:

(1) 进行 SDS -聚丙烯酰胺凝胶电泳(SDS - PAGE),分离胶浓度为 10%,浓缩胶浓度为 4%。

(2) 电泳结束后的凝胶,置于转移缓冲波中平衡 30 min。

(3) 在半干式多用电泳凝胶转移仪进行转膜。

(4) 将转移好的 NC 膜放入脱脂牛奶中 4℃封闭过夜。

(5) 封闭之后的 NC 膜放入 HAA-biotin 中,在 37℃恒温振荡器震荡 2 h。

(6) TTBS 洗涤,10 min 4 次,将 NC 膜放入 HRP - Strep A vitin 中,继续振摇。

(7) TTBS 洗涤,10 min 5 次,将 NC 膜放入 DAB/H_2O_2中,避光显色 5 min。

【结果】

1. ELISA 方法检测 IgA1 异常糖型:加入反应的底物后,底物被催化成为有色产物,产物的量与标本中受检物质的量直接相关,故可根据呈色的深浅进行定性或定量分析。用 405 nm 处吸光度值进行,如果无法检测 405 nm 吸光度值,亦可检测 400~415 nm 范围内的吸光值。

2. Western blotting 方法检测 IgA1 异常糖链:避光显色,由于酶的催化效率很高,间接地放大了免疫反应的结果,显色时间不能过长,显色结果的深浅可反映受检物质的含量。

【注意事项】

凝集素包被酶标板也可在 37℃进行,可使包被时间缩短至 1~2 h。

【思考题】

除了上述方法检测 IgA1 中异常糖链,还有那些免疫学方法可以用来检测 IgA1 中的异常糖链?

(胡艺兰 郭凯文)

Exp. 46   Assay of IgA1 Sugar Chain

【Principle】

There are two subclasses of IgA, IgA1 and IgA2. IgA1 is more prevalent in the serum (and typically monomeric). IgAl is quite extensively glycosylated and has 4 − 5 O-glycosylated sites in the hinge region which is the composition of the O- linked glycan chain. The O- linked glycan chain has the following struction: NeuNAc-Gal-GalNAc-O-Ser(Thr). The abnormal O- linked glycan chain, which lacks terminal Gal and exposes secondary terminal GalNAc, has positive relationship with the pathological symptoms of IgA nephropathy.

According to the principle of specific binding bwtween the lectin and the terminal oligosaccharides, Helix aspersa (HAA), which has the ability of specifically reacting with the terminal GalNAc, can be used to identify the terminal exposing GalNAc in the abnormal lgAl O- linked glycan chain by sandwich ELISA. In addition, biotin agglutinin reaction system can also be applied to detect the abnormal lgAl O- linked glycan chains through Western-bloting.

【Applications】

The appearance of the abnormal serum IgA1 is prior to the clinical symptoms and directly reflects the course of IgA nephropathy, which is closely related to the outcome of therapeutic and prognosis. So the detection of abnormal serum IgA1 is considered to be an ideal method for the diagnosis of IgA nephropathy.

【Materials】

1. Helix aspersa (HAA)
2. Bovine serum albumin(BSA)
3. Anti human IgA antibody labeled alkaline phosphatase (AP)
4. P-nitrophenyl phosphate, disodium(PNPP)
5. PBS
6. PBST: Add Tween − 20 into PBS to the concentration of 0.05%
7. Alkaline phosphatase(AP) buffer (pH9.5), NaCl 5.8 g, MgCl$_2$ 1.0 g, Tris 12.1 g, add three distilled water to constant volume to 1,000 mL
8. TBS: Tris 12.114 g, NaCl 9.00 g, Add tri-distilled water to 1,000 mL, use HCl adjust the pH value to 8, 4℃ preservation
9. 1 mol/L NaOH

10. ELISA reader

11. ELISA plate（bar）

12. Electronic balance

13. Constant temperature water bath

【Procedures】

1. Detection of Abnormal glycan chain in IgAl by ELISA：

（1）Dilute HAA to 5 mg/L with TBS, add 75 μL HAA dilution to each well for coating plate at 4℃ over night.

（2）Wash 4 times with PBST.

（3）Add 200 μL 1% BSA, in 37℃ water bath for 30 min.

（4）Add 75 μL serum without washing, in 37℃ water bath for 2 hours.

（5）Wash 4 times with PBST.

（6）Add 75 μL anti human IgA antibody which labelled AP, in 37℃ water bath for 1 hour.

（7）Wash 5 times with PBST.

（8）Add 75 μL PNPP, in 37℃ water bath for 30 min.

（9）Add 50 μL 1 mol/L NaOH to stop the reaction.

（10）Read OD values in 405 nm by ELISA reader.

2. Detection of Abnormal glycan chain in IgAl by Western blotting：

（1）SDS-polyacrylamide gel electrophoresis（SDS – PAGE）, is carried out by using 10% separation gel and 4% spacer gel.

（2）After electrophoresis, the gel is placed into the transfer buffer solution for 30 minutes.

（3）Transfering in Semi-dry multifunction electrophoretic gel transfer.

（4）Put the transferred NC filter into the skim milk at 4℃ overnight.

（5）After blocking, the NC filter is putted into HAA-biotin, at 37℃ for 2 hours on the constant temperature oscillator.

（6）Wash 4 times with PBST in 10 minutes. Put NC filter into HRP-Strep A vitin and oscillate.

（7）Wash 5 times with PBST in 10 minutes. Put NC filter into DAB/H_2O_2, then observe the result in 5 min in the light shielded environment.

【Results】

1. ELISA method is used to detect IgAl abnormal sugar pattern：after adding the reaction substrate buffer, the substrate buffer is catalyzed to colored products. The amount of the colored products is directly related to the amount of the substance tested in the sample, so it can be qualitatively or quantitatively analyzed according to the color intensity.

2. Detection of abnormal glycan chain in IgAl by Western blotting: light should be avoided for all the color-reaction procedure. Because of the high catalytic efficiency of the enzyme, the result of the immune reaction could be enlarged indirectly. All the coloring time should not be too long. The level of the color shown in the result can reflect the amount of the substance tested in the sample.

【Precautions】

Coating the lectin into ELISA plate can be carried out at 37℃, then the whole coating time can be shortened to 1 − 2 hours.

【Question】

In addition to the above method, what other immunological methods can also be used to detect abnormal the glycan chain in IgA1?

(Hu Yilan　Guo Kaiwen)

实验四十七　细胞表面 N-糖蛋白的代谢标记及检测

【原理】

N-糖蛋白是蛋白质翻译后经过 N-糖基化修饰的蛋白质，主要为分泌蛋白或存在于哺乳动物细胞表面。在细胞培养过程中，在其培养基中添加叠氮修饰的 N-乙酰氨基甘露糖（Ac₄ManNAz），经过细胞摄入、代谢利用，其代谢物叠氮唾液酸（9AzSia）作为糖链成分修饰于翻译后的蛋白质上。叠氮基与二苯基环辛炔荧光染料上的环炔基在一般溶液条件下即可发生 click 反应，进而将荧光标记于细胞表面蛋白 N-糖蛋白上，通过荧光显微镜即可观察到 N-糖蛋白荧光信号（图 47-1）。

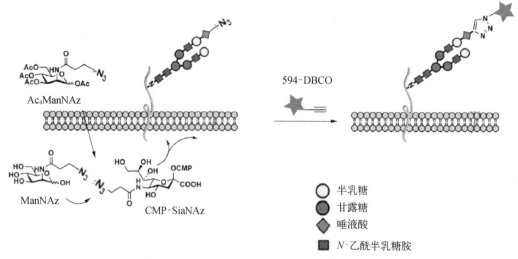

图 47-1　细胞表面 N-糖蛋白的代谢标记示意图

【应用】

可用于观察疾病进展中细胞表面 N-糖基化蛋白糖基化修饰丰度变化或者进行 N-糖基化蛋白共定位研究。

【材料】

1. 叠氮修饰的 N-乙酰氨基甘露糖（Ac₄ManNAz）
2. DMEM 完全培养液（含 10%FBS、1%青霉素—链霉素）
3. PBS
4. 荧光显微镜
5. 二苯基环辛炔荧光染料（594-DBCO）

6. RAW264.7 小鼠巨噬细胞系

7. 0.1% Triton X-100

8. 无菌吸管、CO_2 培养箱、细胞刮子、细胞六孔板

【方法】

1. 细胞培养：提前准备状态较好的 RAW264.7 小鼠巨噬细胞,培养条件为 37℃,5% CO_2。

2. 细胞制备：使用无菌细胞刮子小心地将细胞按照同一顺序刮下来,然后吹散、计数,每个小孔放置 10^6 个细胞,同时添加 50 $\mu mol/L$ 的 $Ac_4ManNAz$,继续培养 3 d,设置不加 $Ac_4ManNAz$ 为对照组。

3. 洗涤：3 天后,弃掉孔内原有的培养液,使用 PBS 洗涤 3 次,每次 3 min。

4. 固定：4%多聚甲醛室温固定 30 min。

5. 洗涤：同步骤 3。

6. 荧光标记：加入 30 $\mu mol/L$ 工作浓度的 594-DBCO,室温放置 30 min。

7. 洗涤：同步骤 3。

8. 结果观察：荧光显微镜观察结果。

【结果】

添加 $Ac_4ManNAz$ 实验组可观察到明显的红色荧光信号,即为 N-糖基化蛋白,而对照组几乎观察不到荧光信号。

【注意事项】

1. 细胞密度不宜过大,一般在 60%~80% 为宜。

2. 细胞培养过程中一定要注意无菌操作。

【思考问题】

细胞内部是否能观察到荧光? 如果能观察到,请解释原因。

（刘传刚　章晓联）

Exp. 47　Metabolic Labelling and Detection of *N*-glycoprotein on Cell Surface

【Principle】

　　N-glycoproteins, modified by *N*-glycosylation after post-translation, are usually presented as secreted proteins or the proteins present on the cellular surface of mammalian cells. For labelling cell-surface *N*-glycoprotein, *N*-azidoacetylmannosamine($Ac_4ManNAz$) is added to the cell culture medium, and then followed by cell uptake and sugar metabolically converted to the corresponding azido sialic acid(9AzSia), which is incorporated into the sialoglycans in a panel of cells. The azide and the alkynyl of diphenylcyclooctyne fluorescent dye (594 − DBCO) can undergo click reaction. The cellular *N*-glycoproteins are labelled fluorescently and can be observed by fluorescence microscopy(Fig.47 − 1).

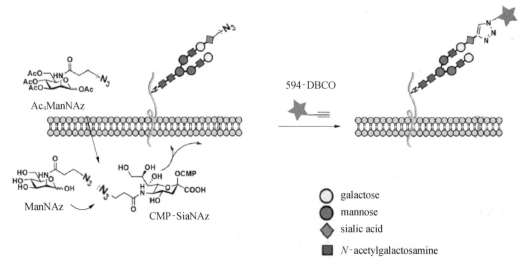

Fig.47 − 1　Schematic illustration of metabolic labeling of cellular surface *N*-glycoprotein

【Application】

　　This experiment can be used to observe changes in cellular protein glycosylation abundance or cellular protein colocalization during disease progression

【Materials】

　　1. N-azidoacetylmannosamine($Ac_4ManNAz$)

　　2. DMEM complete medium containing 10% FBS, 1% penicillin-streptomycin

3. PBS

4. Fluorescence microscope

5. Diphenylcyclooctyne fluorescent dye (594 − DBCO)

6. RAW264. 7 mouse macrophage cell line

7. 0. 1% Triton X − 100

8. Others: sterile pipette, CO_2 incubator, cell scraper, cell 6-well plate

【Procedures】

1. Cell culture: RAW264. 7 mouse macrophages are prepared in advance, culture conditions: 37℃, 5% CO_2.

2. Preparing cells: carefully scrape the cells in the same order using a sterile cell scraper, then blow off and count, place 10^6 cells in each small dish, add 50 μmol /L Ac₄ManNAz, continue to culture for 3d. Set no Ac₄ManNAz as control group.

3. Washing: after 3 days, the original medium in the small dish is discarded and cells are washed three times with PBS, 3 min/time.

4. Fixation: add 4% paraformaldehyde to fix cells at room temperature for 30 min.

5. Wash: same as 3.

6. Fluorescent labelling: Add 594 − DBCO at a working concentration of 30 μmol /L and leave it at room temperature for 30 min.

7. Wash: same as 3.

8. Results observation: observe the fluorescence under fluorescence microscope.

【Results】

A significant red fluorescence signal can be observed in the experimental group supplemented with Ac₄ManNAz, while no fluorescence signal is observed in the control group.

【Precautions】

1. Cell density should not be too high, generally 60%−80% cell density is appropriate.

2. Be sure to pay attention to aseptic operation during cell culture.

【Question】

Can you observe fluorescence inside of the cell? If you can, what is the reason for it?

(Liu Chuangang Zhang Xiaolian)

实验四十八　胞内 O-GlcNAc 糖蛋白的标记及检测

【原理】

细胞内 O-GlcNAc 糖蛋白存在于细胞核和细胞质中,蛋白质翻译后在 O-糖基化转移酶(O-GlcNAc transferase,OGT)的催化下将 UDP-GlcNAc 中的 GlcNAc 基团连接到底物蛋白的丝氨酸或苏氨酸的羟基上,该底物蛋白即为 O-GlcNAc 糖蛋白。在细胞培养过程中,经过细胞摄入叠氮基修饰的 N-乙酰葡萄糖代谢利用,在 OGT 的催化下将 HBP 代谢途径的产物 UDP-GlcNAz 中的 GlcNAz 基团连接到底物蛋白的丝氨酸或苏氨酸的羟基上。叠氮基与二苯基环辛炔荧光染料上的炔基在一般溶液条件下即可发生点击反应,进而将荧光标记于 O-GlcNAc 糖蛋白上,通过荧光显微镜可以观察到蛋白荧光信号(图 48-1)。

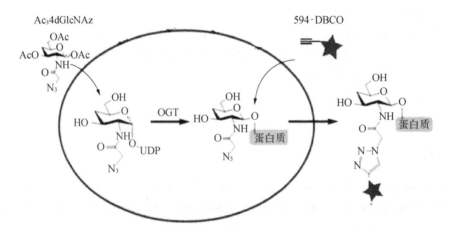

图 48-1　细胞内 O-GlcNAc 糖蛋白的代谢标记示意图

【应用】

可用于观察疾病进展中细胞 O-GlcNAc 糖蛋白糖基化丰度变化或者进行蛋白共定位研究。

【材料】

1. 叠氮基修饰的 N-乙酰氨基葡萄糖(4-脱氧)(Ac₃4dGlcNAz)
2. DMEM 完全培养液(含 10%FBS、1%青霉素-链霉素)
3. PBS
4. 荧光显微镜
5. 二苯基环辛炔荧光染料(594-DBCO)

6. RAW264. 7 小鼠巨噬细胞系

7. 0. 1% Triton X - 100

8. 无菌吸管、二氧化碳培养箱、细胞刮子、细胞六孔板

【方法】

1. 细胞培养：提前准备好 RAW264. 7 小鼠巨噬细胞，培养条件为 37℃、5%CO$_2$。

2. 细胞制备：使用无菌细胞刮子小心地将细胞按照同一顺序刮下来，然后吹散、计数，每个孔内放置 10^6 个细胞，同时添加 50 μmol/L 的 Ac$_3$4dGlcNAz，继续培养 3 d，设置不加 Ac$_3$4dGlcNAz 的对照组。

3. 洗涤：3 天后，弃掉孔内原有的培养液，使用 PBS 洗涤 3 次，每次 3 min。

4. 固定：4% 多聚甲醛室温固定 30 min。

5. 洗涤：同步骤 3。

6. 破膜：使用含 0. 1% Triton-100 PBS 室温孵育 10 min。

7. 洗涤：同步骤 3。

8. 荧光标记：加入 30 μmol/L 的工作浓度的 594 - DBCO，室温放置 30 min。

9. 洗涤：同步骤 3。

10. 结果观察：荧光显微镜观察结果。

【结果】

添加 Ac$_3$4dGlcNAz 实验组可观察到明显的红色荧光信号，即为标记的细胞内 O - GlcNAc 修饰的糖蛋白，而对照组几乎观察不到荧光信号。

【注意事项】

1. 细胞密度不宜过大，一般在 60%~80% 为宜。

2. 严格控制破膜时间。

3. 细胞培养过程中一定要注意无菌操作。

【思考问题】

实验中采用 Triton X - 100 的目的是什么？

（刘传刚　章晓联）

Exp. 48   Metabolic Labelling and Detection of Intracellular O – GlcNAc glycoprotein

【Principle】

The intracellular O – GlcNAc glycoprotein is present in the nucleus and cytoplasm, and the GlcNAc from UDP – GlcNAc is linked to the serine or threonine of the protein under the catalysis of O – GlcNAc transferase (OGT). For labelling intracellular O – GlcNAc glycoprotein, the 1, 3, 6 – tri – O – acetyl – 2 – azidoacetamido – 2, 4 – dideoxy – D – glucopyranose (Ac$_3$4dGlcNAz) is added to the cell culture medium for cell metabolism, and the GlcNAz group in the product UDP – GlcNAz of the HBP metabolic pathway is linked to the serine or threonine of the substrate protein under the catalysis of OGT. The azide and the alkynyl can undergo click reaction under normal solution conditions, and then the O – GlcNAc glycoproteins are labelled fluorescently, and the fluorescence signal of O – GlcNAc glycoproteins can be observed by fluorescence microscopy (Fig.48 – 1).

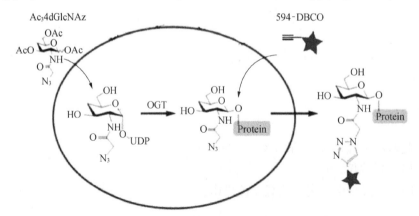

Fig.48 – 1   Schematic illustration of metabolic labeling of intracellular O – GlcNAc glycoprotein

【Application】

It can be used to observe changes of O – GlcNAc glycosylation abundance or cellular O – GlcNAc colocalization during disease progression

【Materials】

1. 1,3,6 – tri – O – acetyl – 2 – azidoacetamido – 2,4 – dideoxy – D – glucopyranose (Ac$_3$4dGlcNAz)

2. DMEM complete medium containing 10% FBS, 1% penicillin-streptomycin

3. PBS

4. Fluorescence microscope

5. Diphenylcyclooctyne fluorescent dye (594 - DBCO)

6. RAW264. 7 mouse macrophage cell line

7. 0. 1% Triton X - 100

8. sterile pipette, CO_2 incubator, cell scraper, cell 6-well plate

【Procedures】

1. Cell culture: RAW264. 7 mouse macrophages are prepared in advance, culture conditions: 37℃, 5% CO_2.

2. Preparing cells: carefully scrape the cells in the same order using a sterile cell scraper, then blow off and count, place 10^6 cells in each small dish, add 50 μmol/L Ac$_3$4dGlcNAz, continue to culture for 3d. , set no Ac$_3$4dGlcNAz as control group.

3. Washing: after 3 days, discard the original medium in the small dish was and washed plates three times with PBS, 3 min/time.

4. Fixation: 4% paraformaldehyde is added to fix cells at room temperature for 30 min.

5. Wash: the same as 3.

6. Permeabilization: incubate cells for 10 min at room temperature with 0. 1% Triton-100 PBS.

7. Wash: the same as 3.

8. Fluorescent labelling: add 594 - DBCO at a working concentration of 30 μmol/L and leave it at room temperature for 30 min.

9. Wash: same as 3.

10. Results observation: observe the fluorescence with fluorescence microscope.

【Results】

A significant red fluorescence signal can be observed in the experimental group supplemented with Ac$_3$4dGlcNAz, while no fluorescence signal is observed in the control group.

【Precautions】

1. Cell density should not be too high, generally 60%- 80% is appropriate.

2. Strictly control the permeabilization time.

3. Be sure to pay attention to aseptic operation during cell culture.

【Question】

What is the purpose of using 0. 1% Triton-100 in the experiment?

(Liu Chuangang   Zhang Xiaolian)

主要参考文献
References

高东花,张铭珺,朱劲涛.人工荨麻疹患者尘螨特异性 IgE 与总 IgE 水平分析.中国实用医药,2018,13(16):99-100.

何维,曹雪涛,熊思冬,等.医学免疫学.第二版.北京:人民卫生出版社,2014:129-131.

科利根 JE,比勒 BE,马吉利斯 DH,等.精编免疫学实验指南.曹雪涛等译.北京:科学出版社,2009:31.

刘辉,朱正美.简明免疫学技术.北京:科学出版社,2002:239-241.

卢传林.过敏原特异性 IgE 检测在过敏性鼻炎患儿中的应用意义.白求恩医学杂志,2016,14(2):238-239.

司传平.医学免疫学实验.北京:人民卫生出版社,2005:48.

谭宁,贺守第,倪慧婕,等.类风湿关节炎血清植物性食物过敏原特异性 IgG 和 IgE 检测.中华临床免疫和变态反应杂志,2016,2(4):97-100.

张波,许继宗,李玉华,等.变应性鼻炎患者血清 IgE 及嗜酸性粒细胞的季节变化研究.世界中医药,2014,9(10):1313-1315.

章晓联.免疫学及实验技术新进展.北京:中华医学电子音像出版社,2018:21-25.

Abel AM, Yang C, Thakar MS, et al. Natural killer cells: development, maturation, and clinical utilization. Frontiers in Immunology, 2018,9: 1869.

Brandtzaeg P, Kiyono H, Pabst R, et al. Terminology: nomenclature of mucosa-associated lymphoid tissue. Mucosal Immunology, 2008,1: 31-7.

Du C, Xie X. G protein-coupled receptors as therapeutic targets for multiple sclerosis. Cell Research, 2012,22: 1108-1128.

Duellman SJ, Valley MP, Kotraiah V, et al. A bioluminescence assay for aldehyde dehydrogenase activity. Analytical Biochemistry, 2013,434: 226-232.

Ebioscience. Intracellular immunofluorescent staining for flow cytometric analysis (FACS analysis).2009. http://diyhpl.us/~bryan/irc/protocol-online/protocol-cache/FCI.htm [2018-8-25].

Foster B, Prussin C, Liu F, et al. Detection of intracellular cytokines by flow cytometry. Current Protocols in Immunology, 2007, 78.

Hackett J, Tutt M, Lipscomb M, et al. Origin and differentiation of natural killer cells. II. Functional and morphologic studies of purified NK-1.1+cells. J Immunol, 1986,136: 3124-3131.

Hietanen T, Pitkanen M, Kapanen M, et al. Post-irradiation viability and cytotoxicity of natural killer cells isolated from human peripheral blood using different methods. International Journal of Radiation Biology, 2016,92: 71-79.

Jahr H, Pfeiffer G, Hering BJ, et al. Endotoxin-mediated activation of cytokine production in human PBMCs by collagenase and Ficoll. J Mol Med (Berl),1999, 77: 118-120.

Jiang H, English BP, Hazan RB, et al. Tracking surface glycans on live cancer cells with single-molecule sensitivity. Angew Chem Int Ed Engl,2015,54: 1765-1769.

Kim SB, Naganawa R, Murata S, et al. A bioluminescence assay system for imaging metal cationic activities in urban aerosols. Methods Mol Biol,2016,1461: 279－287.

Li J, Wang J, Wen L, et al. An OGA－resistant probe allows specific visualization and accurate identification of O－GlcNAc－modified proteins in cells. ACS Chemical Biology, 2016, 11: 3002－3006.

Li X, Meng M, Zheng L, et al. Chemiluminescence immunoassay for S-adenosylhomocysteine detection and its application in DNA methyltransferase activity evaluation and inhibitors screening. Analytical Chemistry, 2016,88: 8556－8561.

Liu KK, Wang QT, Yang SM, et al. Ginsenoside compound K suppresses the abnormal activation of T lymphocytes in mice with collagen-induced arthritis. Acta Pharmacologica Sinica, 2014, 35: 599－612.

Lomakina GY, Modestova YA, Ugarova NN. Bioluminescence assay for cell viability. Biochemistry. Biokhimiia, 2015,80: 701－713.

Lu LL, Chung AW, Rosebrock TR, et al. A Functional role for antibodies in tuberculosis. Cell, 2016, 167: 433－443.

Marim FM, Silveira TN, Lima DS, et al. A method for generation of bone marrow-derived macrophages from cryopreserved mouse bone marrow cells. PloS One, 2010, 5: e15263.

Martinet L, Ferrari De Andrade L, Guillerey C, et al. DNAM－1 expression marks an alternative program of NK cell maturation. Cell Reports, 2015, 11: 85－97.

Nakano H, Cook DN. Pulmonary antigen presenting cells: isolation, purification, and culture. Methods Mol Biol, 2013,1032: 19－29.

Park HR, Hwang D, Suh HJ, et al. Antitumor and antimetastatic activities of rhamnogalacturonan-II-type polysaccharide isolated from mature leaves of green tea via activation of macrophages and natural killer cells. International Journal of Biological Macromolecules, 2017, 99: 179－186.

Stromnes IM, Goverman JM. Active induction of experimental allergic encephalomyelitis. Nature Protocols, 2006,1: 1810－1819.

Sun Y, Chen H, Dai J, et al. HMGB1 expression patterns during the progression of experimental autoimmune encephalomyelitis. Journal of Neuroimmunology, 2015, 280: 29－35.

Weischenfeldt J, Porse B. Bone marrow-derived macrophages (BMM): isolation and applications. CSH Protocols, 2008,2008: pdb prot5080.

Wen L, Zheng Y, Jiang K, et al. Two-step chemoenzymatic detection of *N*-acetylneuraminic acid-alpha (2－3)－galactose glycans. Journal of the American Chemical Society, 2016, 138: 11473－11476.

Yang Z, Cao Y, Li J, et al. A new label-free strategy for a highly efficient chemiluminescence immunoassay. Chem Commun (Camb), 2015,51: 14443－14446.

Yuan Y, Xu S, Cheng X, et al. Bioorthogonal turn-On probe based on aggregation-induced emission characteristics for cancer cell imaging and ablation. Angew Chem Int Ed Engl, 2016, 55: 6457 – 6461.

附录

Appendices

附录一　　常用试剂和培养液

【抗凝剂】

1. 500 U/mL 肝素溶液：取 1 支 12 500 U 的肝素注射液，用无菌生理盐水稀释 25 倍，即为 500 U/mL。4℃保存。使用时取 0.1 mL 可抗凝血 2 mL。

2. Alsever's 保存液：

柠檬酸三钠·2H$_2$O	0.8 g
柠檬酸	0.055 g
NaCl	0.42 g
葡萄糖	2.05 g
双蒸水	100 mL

将各成分溶解后，用滤纸过滤，分装，112.6℃灭菌 30 min，4℃保存。取血时按 1∶1 比例与新鲜血液混合。

【染色剂】

1. 1%美蓝染液：

美蓝	1 g
0.9%NaCl	100 mL

溶解后，过滤。

2. 姬姆萨-瑞氏染液：

瑞氏染料粉	0.3 g
姬姆萨粉	0.03 g
甲醇	100 mL

将 2 种粉末置研钵中研细，再逐滴加入甲醇，混匀后倒入棕色瓶中。充分振摇，置室温溶解后使用。

3. 0.5%台盼蓝染液：

（1）台盼蓝染料	1 g
蒸馏水	100 mL

将染料置研钵内边研磨边加蒸馏水溶解。

（2）NaCl	1.7 g
蒸馏水	100 mL

临用前取（1）、（2）液等量混合，离心沉淀，取上清供染色用。

4. Hoechst33342 染液：用 PBS 配成 10 mg/mL 的储存液，避光保存于 4℃。

5. 考马斯亮蓝染液：1%考马斯亮蓝 R250（40%甲醇，10% 乙酸）。

【缓冲液和试剂】

1. 磷酸盐缓冲液(pH 7.4):

K_2HPO_4	1.392 g
$NaH_2PO \cdot H_2O$	0.276 g
NaCl	8.770 g

先溶于 900 mL 蒸馏水,然后用 0.01 mol/L KOH 调 pH 至 7.4,用蒸馏水定容到 1 000 mL。

2. 磷酸缓冲盐溶液(PBS),10×和1×:

10×储存液,1 000 mL:	1× 工作液,pH 7.3:
80 g NaCl	137 mmol/L NaCl
2 g KCl	2.7 mmol/L KCl
11.5 g $NaHPO_4.7H_2O$	4.3 mmol/L $NaHPO_4 \cdot 7H_2O$
2 g KH_2PO_4	1.4 mmol/L KH_2PO_4

3. TE 缓冲液:

0.1 mol/L Tris-HCl

10 mmol/L EDTA, pH 8.0

4. 50×TAE 电泳缓冲液:

Tris 碱	242 g
冰醋酸	57.1 mL
0.5 mmol/L EDTA,pH 8.0	100 mL

加蒸馏水定容至 1 000 mL。

5. 6×凝胶加样缓冲液:

0.25%溴酚蓝

40%蔗糖

加水溶解,4℃保存。

6. 1.5 mol/L pH 8.8 Tris-HCl 分离胶缓冲液:

Tris	18.2 g
SDS	0.4 g

HCl 调 pH 至 8.8,总体积为 100 mL。

7. 0.5 mol/L pH 6.8 Tris-HCl 浓缩胶缓冲液:

Tris	6.05 g
SDS	0.4 g

HCl 调至 6.8,总体积为 100 mL。

8. 0.05 mol/L Tris-甘氨酸电极缓冲液:

Tris	15 g
Gly	72 g
SDS	5 g

加水至 500 mL(临用时稀释 10 倍)。

9. 0.025 mol/L pH 8.3 转移电极缓冲液:

Tris	3.785 g
Gly	19.3 g

加水至 1 000 mL,溶解后加甲醇溶液 200 mL。

10. 洗涤缓冲液:

TBS pH7.6 (1 L 体积中含有 2.42 g Tris base, 8 g NaCl, 4 mL 1mol/L HCl)

TBST [TBS 含有 0.1%(m/V) Tween-20]

11. 封被液:TBS 含有 10%(m/V)去脂奶粉, 0.1% Tween-20。

12. 2×SDS 凝胶加样缓冲液:

100 mmol/L Tris-HCl,pH 6.8

200 mmol/L 二硫苏糖醇(DTT)

4% SDS,0.2% 溴酚蓝

20%甘油

不含 DTT 的 2×SDS 凝胶加样缓冲液可保存于室温,临用前须从-20℃储存的 1 mmol/L DTT 储存液取出适量现加入上述缓冲液中。200 mmol/L DTT 可用 1.5% 2-ME 代替。

13. 红细胞裂解缓冲液:

0.32 mL 蔗糖

1%(V/V)Triton X-100

5 mol/L $MgCl_2$

12 mmol/L Tris-HCl, pH7.5

14. 白细胞裂解缓冲液:pH 8.0

10 mmol/L Tris-HCl

10 mmol/L NaCl

10 mmol/L EDTA

1% SDS

15. 0.05 mol/L 巴比妥缓冲液,pH 8.6:

巴比妥钠	10.3 g
巴比妥	1.84 g
蒸馏水	加至 1 000 mL

16. 0.4%巴比妥琼脂:

琼脂粉	0.4 g
巴比妥缓冲液	100 mL

加热溶解琼脂粉,4℃保存备用。

17. 3%巴比妥琼脂:

琼脂粉	3 g
巴比妥缓冲液	100 mL

加热溶解琼脂粉,4℃保存备用。

18. Hank's 平衡盐溶液:

储存液: A 液(1) NaCl   80 g

KCl	4 g
$MgSO_4 \cdot 7H_2O$	1 g
$MgCl_2 \cdot 6 H_2O$	1 g
双蒸水加至	450 mL
(2) $CaCl_2$	1.4 g
双蒸水加至	50 mL

将(1)(2)液混合,112.6℃灭菌 15 min,4℃保存。

B 液(1)$Na_2HPO_4 \cdot 12H_2O$	1.52 g
KH_2PO_4	0.60 g
葡萄糖	10 g
双蒸水加至	400 mL
(2) 0.4%酚红溶液	100 mL

将(1)(2)液混合,112.6℃灭菌 15 min,4℃保存。

应用液:A 液 25 mL+B 液 25 mL+双蒸水 450 mL,112.6℃灭菌 15 min,4℃保存。可用 1 个月。使用前用 $NaHCO_3$ 调 pH 至 7.2~7.4。

19. 无 Ca^{2+}、Mg^{2+} Hank's 液:

储存液: NaCl	80 g
KCl	4 g
$Na_2HPO_4 \cdot 12H_2O$	1.52 g
KH_2PO_4	0.60 g
葡萄糖	10 g

加双蒸水使各组分溶解后,加入 0.4%酚红溶液 50 mL,再加双蒸水至 1 000 mL。4℃保存。

应用液:将原液用双蒸水作 1∶10 稀释,112.6℃灭菌 15 min,4℃保存。可用 1 个月。使用前用无菌 $NaHCO_3$ 调 pH 至 7.2~7.4。

20. Earle's 液:

A 液(10×):

NaCl	68 g
KCl	4 g
$NaH_2PO_4 \cdot H_2O$	1.4 g
$MgSO_4 \cdot 7H_2O$	2 g
葡萄糖	10 g
双蒸水	800 mL
10%酚红	10 mL

上述各项逐一溶解后加双蒸水至 1 000 mL。

B 液(100×):

$CaCl_2$	2 g
双蒸水	100 mL

A 液和 B 液分别经 116℃ 15 min 灭菌,4℃ 保存。

应用液:

A 液	100 mL
B 液	10 mL
双蒸水	890 mL

21. 0.8% 戊二醛:

25% 戊二醛	0.8 mL
0.43% NaCl	24.2 mL

临用前配制。

22. 细胞裂解液:

10 mmol/L Tris-HCl,pH 8.0

10 mmol/L NaCl

10 mmol/L EDTA

100 μg/mL 蛋白酶 K

1% SDS

23. 6 mol/L NaI:90 g NaI,加蒸馏水,溶解定容至 100 mL, 高压灭菌。

24. 3 mol/L 醋酸钠:408.1 g NaAC · $3H_2O$,溶于 800 mL 蒸馏水,用冰醋酸调节 pH 至 5.2,然后蒸馏水定容到 1 000 mL。

25. 碘化丙啶(PI)溶液:溶解 100 mg PI 于 10 mL 去离子水中,避光保存于 4℃ 中。

26. 30% 聚丙烯酰胺(30% Acr/Bis):

丙烯酰胺(Acr)	29 g
N,N'-亚甲双丙烯酰胺(Bis)	1 g

加水至 100 mL。室温避光保存数月。

27. 10% 过硫酸铵(APS):过硫酸铵 1 g,加水至 10 mL。4℃ 保存数周。

28. 浓缩胶配方:

30% Acr/Bis	0.666 mL
H_2O	3.033 mL
10% APS	0.25 mL

29. 10% 十二烷基硫酸钠(SDS):用去离子水配制成 10% 储存液,保存于室温。

30. PCR 混合液:

5'端和 3'端的引物	2 pmol
内参照引物(β-actin 基因引物)	2 pmol
各种 d-NTP(dATP,dCTP,dGTP,dTTP)	200 μmol
Taq 多聚酶(终浓度为 1%~2%, U/μL)	

1×PCR 缓冲液:10 mmol/L Tris-HCl(pH8.3), 50 mmol/L KCl, 1.5 mmol/L $MgCl_2$,

0.01%明胶

　　Ficoll 400（终浓度为 1%，V/V）

　　加样缓冲液（甲酚红，终浓度为 0.001%，m/V）

　　上述引物混合液准备好后,分装至作好标记的 PCR 扩增管中,每管 38 μL,反应终体积为 40 μL。反应体积的调整使用双蒸水,不要使用 TE, ETDA 可抑制 *Taq* 多聚酶的活性。置于−20℃保存,临用时取出。

　　31. 闪烁液的配制:将 PPO(2,5 -二苯基噁唑)4.0 g,POPOP[1,4 -双-2 -(5 -苯基噁唑)]0.2 g 加入二甲苯(A.R.)1 000 mL 中混合,置 70~80℃水浴箱中轻轻摇匀,充分溶解后备用。

　　32. 聚己二醇溶液的配制:将 50 g PEG 加入热的 PBS(置 37℃水浴箱)中,调至 100 mL。分装于 10 mL 玻璃瓶,每瓶 5 mL,经 120℃ 15 min 高压灭菌。于 4℃储存备用。

【培养液】

　　1. RPMI - 1640 培养液:

RPMI - 1640 干粉	10.4 g
Hepes	5.95 g
三蒸水加至	1 000 mL

摇匀,置 4℃过夜,使其完全溶解。过滤除菌,分装并置−20℃保存,可供 6 月使用。

　　2. RPMI - 1640 完全培养液:

RPMI - 1640 培养液	170 mL
胎牛血清	20 mL
青霉素(100 000 U/mL)	2 mL
链霉素(10 000 mg/mL)	2 mL
L -谷氨酰胺(200 mmol/L)	2 mL

混匀,用 $NaHCO_3$ 溶液调 pH 至 7.1 左右,过滤除菌,−20℃以下保存。

　　3. 淋巴细胞培养液:含有 50 μg/mL 庆大霉素及 10% FCS 的 RPMI - 1640(GIBCO),4℃保存。

　　4. HAT 储存液的配制

　　(1) 100 倍浓缩的次黄嘌呤和胸腺嘧啶核苷(HT)储存液:将 136.1 mg 次黄嘌呤(分子量 136.1 Da)和 38.8 mg 胸腺嘧啶核苷(分子量 242.2 Da)加入 100 mL 双蒸水(置于 50℃)中。用滤膜过滤除菌,以每瓶 2~5 mL 储存于−20℃。

　　(2) 100 倍浓缩的氨基蝶呤储存液:将 1.76 mg 氨基蝶呤(分子量 440.4 Da)加入90 mL 双蒸水中。逐滴加入 1 mol/L NaOH,直到氨基蝶呤溶解,再用 1 mol/L HCl 调 pH 至 7.5。用双蒸水将终体积调至 100 mL。用滤膜过滤除菌,以每瓶 2~5 mL 储存于−20℃。

　　5. HAT 培养液的配制:取 HT 储存液和 A 储存液各 2 mL 加入 96 mL 含 10% 血清的组织培养液中。

（章晓联）

Appendice 1　Commonly Used Reagents and Media

【Anticoagulants】

1. 500 U/mL heparin solutions: take a heparin injection containing 12 500 U and dilute 25 times with 0.9% sterile saline solution. Store at 4℃. 500 U/mL of 0.1mL heparin solution may be used to resist 2 mL blood to clot.

2. Alsever's preservative solution:

Sodium citrate · 2H$_2$O	0.8 g
Citrate	0.055 g
NaCl	0.42 g
Glucose	2.05 g
Distilled water	100 mL

Dissolve each component in distilled water. Pass through a filter paper. Sterilize at 112.6℃ for 30 min. Store at 4℃. To use, mix with fresh blood in proportion of 1 : 1.

【Staining solutions】

1. 1% methylene blue staining solution:

Methylene blue	1 g
0.9% NaCl	100 mL

Dissolve and filtrate

2. Giemsa-Wright staining solution:

Wright powder	0.3 g
Giemsa powder	0.03 g
Methanol	100 mL

Powders are crushed in mortar with a pestle while adding methanol. Place into a brown bottle. Shake well. Dissolve at room temperature to use.

3. 0.5% Trypan blue staining solution:

(1) Trypan blue	1 g
Distilled water	100 mL

Stains are crushed in mortar with a pestle while adding distilled water to dissolve them.

(2) NaCl	1.7 g
Distilled water	100 mL

Before using, mix (1) with (2) using an equal volume. Centrifuge and precipitate. Take the supernatant for the use of staining.

4. Hoechst33342 dyes: prepared as 10 μg/mL stock solution with PBS. Keep in the dark at 4℃.

5. Coomassie Brilliant Blue Staining buffer: 1% Coomassie Brilliant Blue R250 (40% MeOH, 10% HOAC).

【Buffers and reagents】

1. Phosphate-buffered saline (PBS, pH 7.4):

100 mmol/L NaCl

20 mmol/L NaH_2PO_4

80 mmol/L Na_2HPO_4

2. PBS buffer, 10× and 1×:

10× stock solution, 1 000 mL: 1× working solution, pH 7.3:

80 g NaCl   137 mmol/L NaCl

2 g KCl   2.7 mmol/L KCl

11.5 g $NaHPO_4 \cdot 7H_2O$ 4.3 mmol/L $NaHPO_4 \cdot 7H_2O$

2 g KH_2PO_4 1.4 mmol/L KH_2PO_4

3. TE buffer:

0.1mol/L Tris-HCl, pH8.0

10 mmol/L EDTA

4. 50×TAE electrophoresis buffer:

Tris-base   242 g

ice HAC   57.1 mL

0.5 mmol/L EDTA pH 8.0   100 mL

Final volume is 1 000 mL.

5. 6×gel loading buffers: 0.25%, 40% sucrose; dissolved in dH_2O, store at 4℃.

6. 1.5 mol/L pH 6.8 Tris-HCl separate gel buffer:

Tris   18.2 g

SDS   0.4 g

Adjusting pH to 8.8 with HCl, final volume is 100 mL.

7. 0.5 mol/L pH 6.8 Tris-HCl stacking gel buffer:

Tris   6.05 g

SDS   0.4 g

Adjusting pH to 6.8 with HCl, final volume is 100mL.

8. 0.05 mol/L Tris-Glycine electrode buffer (diluted 10 times when using):

Tris   15 g

Glycine   72 g

SDS   5 g

Adding dH_2O to final 500 mL.

9. 0.025 mol/L pH 8.3 electro blotting buffer：

Tris	3.785 g
Glycine	19.3 g

Dissolved in dH$_2$O, add 200 mL methanol, final volume 1 000 mL.

10. Wash buffer：

TBS pH 7.6 (1 L containing 2.42 g Tris base, 8 g NaCl, 4 mL1 mol/L HCl)

TBST [TBS with 0.1% (m/V) Tween-20]

11. Blocking buffer：TBS containing 10% (m/V) non-fat milk, 0.1% Tween-20.

12. 2×SDS gel loading buffer：

100 mmol/L Tris-HCl, pH 6.8

200 mmol/L DTT

4% SDS, 0.2% bromoblue

20% glycerol

13. RBC lysis buffer：

0.3 mol/L sucrose

1%(V/V) Triton X-100

5 mmol/L MgCl$_2$

12 mmol/L Tris-HCl, pH7.5

14. WBC lysis buffer：

10 mmol/L Tris-HCl, pH8.0,

10 mmol/L NaCl

10 mmol/L EDTA

1%SDS

15. 0.05 mol/L barbital buffer, pH 8.6：

Sodium barbital	1.03 g
Barbital	1.84 g

Add distilled water up to 1 000 mL.

16. 0.4% barbital agar：

Agar powder	0.4 g
Barbital buffer	100 mL

Heat to dissolve agar powder and store at 4℃ before the reagent used.

17. 3% barbital agar：

Agar powder	3 g
Barbital buffer	100 mL

Heat to dissolve agar powder and store at 4℃ before the reagent used.

18. Hank's balanced salt solution (HBSS)：

Store solution：solution A (1) NaCl	80 g
KCl	4 g

MgSO$_4$ · 7H$_2$O	1 g
MgCl$_2$ · 6H$_2$O	1 g
Distilled water add up to	450 mL
(2) CaCl$_2$	1.4 g
Distilled water add up to	50 mL

Mix (1) with (2) and sterilize at 112.6 ℃ for 15 min. Store at 4℃.

Solution B (1) Na$_2$HPO$_4$ · 12 H$_2$O	1.52 g
K$_2$HPO$_4$	0.60 g
Glucose	10 g
Distilled water add up to	400 mL
(2) 0.4% phenol red solution	100 mL

Mix (1) with (2) and sterilize at 112.6 ℃ for 15 min. Store at 4℃.

Work solution: Take A solution 25 mL, B solution 25 mLand distilled water 450 mL and sterilize at 112.6 ℃ for 15 min. Store at 4℃. It may be used up to one month. Before using, adjust pH to 7.2 − 7.4 with NaHCO$_3$ solution.

19. Ca^{++}-and Mg^{++}-free Hank's Balanced Salt Solution:

Store solution: NaCl	80 g
KCl	4 g
Na$_2$HPO$_4$ · 12 H$_2$O	1.52 g
K$_2$HPO$_4$	0.60 g
Glucose	10 g

Dissolve each component in distilled water. Add 50 mL of 0.4% phenol red. Distilled water add up to 1 000 mL. Store at 4℃.

Work solution: Dilute store solution to 1 : 10 with distilled water. Sterilize at 112.6 ℃ for 15 min. Store at 4℃. May be used up to 1 month. Before using, adjust pH to 7.2 − 7.4 with NaHCO$_3$ solution.

20. Earle's solution:

Solution A (10×):

NaCl	68 g
KCl	4 g
NaH$_2$PO$_4$ · H$_2$O	1.4 g
MgSO$_4$ · 7H$_2$O	2 g
Glucose	10 g
Twice-distilled water	800 mL
10% Phenol Red	10 mL

After above various components being dissolved one by one, add twice-distilled water to 1 000 mL.

Solution B (100×):

| CaCl$_2$ | 2 g |
| Twice-distilled water | 100 mL |

Autoclave solution A and B at 116℃ for 15 min respectively and then store at 4℃.

Applicative solution:

Solution A	100 mL
Solution B	10 mL
Twice-distilled water	890 mL

21. 0.8% glutaraldehyde water solution:

| 25% glutaraldehyde | 0.8 mL |
| 0.43% NaCl | 24.2 mL |

Prepare prior to use.

22. Cell lystaes:

10 mmol/L Tris-HCl, pH8.0

10 mmol/L NaCl

10 mmol/L EDTA

100 g/mL proteinase K

1% SDS

23. 6 mol/L NaI: 90 g NaI dissolved in dH$_2$O, final volume is 100 mL, and can be sterile by autoclave.

24. 3 mol/L NaAc: 408.1 g NaAc · 3H$_2$O dissolved in dH$_2$O, ice HAC adjust pH to 5.2, final volume is 1 000 mL.

25. Propidium iodide (PI) solution: dissolve 10 mg of propidium iodide in 10 mL distilled water. Store at 4℃ in the dark.

26. 30% Acrylamide/Bis:

| Acrylamide | 29 g |
| Bis | 1 g |

Dissolved in dH$_2$O, final volume is 100 mL, store at room temperature in dark for several months.

27. 10% ammonium persulfate (APS) (m/V): 1 g APS dissolved in dH$_2$O, final volume is 10 mL.

28. Stacking gel:

30% Acr/Bis	0.666 mL
H$_2$O	3.033 mL
10% APS	0.25 mL

29. 10% SDS (m/V): 10 g SDS dissolved in dH$_2$O, final volume is 10 mL.

30. PCR mixture (containing HLA－B27 SSP, Taq enzyme, dNTP, internal positive reference primers, etc.):

5′ primer and 3′ primer of HLA－B27 gene　　　　　　　　　　2 pmol

internal positive reference primers(5′ primer and 3′ primer of β – actin gene)   2 pmol

dNTP (dATP, dCTP, dGTP, dTTP)   200 μmol

Taq enzyme(final concentration 1%– 2%, U/μL)

1×PCR buffer: 10 mmol/L Tris-HCl, pH8.3, 50 mmol/L KCl, 1.5 mmol/L $MgCl_2$, 0.01% gelatin

Ficoll 400 (final concentration 1%, V/V)

Loading buffer(cresol red,final concentration 0.001%, m/V)

After the preparation of the PCR mixture, aliquot it to several PCR tubes, 38 μL for each tube, and the final volume for amplification is 40 μL. Using dd H_2O to adjust the amplification volume, and do not use the TE solution, for the TE is able to inhibit the activity of the Taq polymerase. The aliquot should be kept at $-20℃$ for storage, and thaw before use.

31. Preparation of scintillation liquid: mix PPO (2,5 – diphenyloxazole) 4.0 g, POPOP [1,4 – Bis – 2 –(5 – phenyloxazole)] 0.2 g in 1 000 mL dimethyl benzene (A.R.) and shake slightly in $70 – 80℃$ water bath to dissolve completely for use.

32. Preparation of polyethylene glycol solution: add 50 g PEG to warm PBS (in a 37℃ water bath) and adjust to 100 mL. Dispense 5 mL aliquots into 10 mL glass bottles and autoclave at 120℃ 15 min. Store at 4℃ for use.

【Media】

1. RPMI – 1640 medium:

RPMI – 1640 powder	10.4 g
Hepes	5.95 g
Distilled water add up to	1 000 mL

Mix well. Store at 4℃ for overnight to completely dissolve powder. Filter to sterilize. Store at $-20℃$. It may be used up 6 months.

2. RPMI – 1640 complete medium:

RPMI – 1640 medium	170 mL
Fetal calf serum	20 mL
Penicillin (10 000 U/mL)	2 mL
Streptomycin (10 000 mg/mL)	2 mL
L-glutamine (200 mmol/L)	2 mL

Mix well. Adjust pH to 7.1 using $NaHCO_3$ solution. Filter to sterilize. Store at $-20℃$.

3. Lymphocyte culture medium (LCM):

RPMI – 1640 (GIBCO) containing:	50 μg/mL gentamicin
	10% FCS

Store up to 2 weeks at 4℃.

4. Preparation of HAT stock solution

(1) 100 – fold concentrated stock solution of hypoxanthine and thymidine (HT):

dissolve 136.1 mg hypoxanthine (molecular weight 136.1 Da) and 38.8 mg thymidine (molecular weight 242.2 Da) in 100 mL twice-distilled water at 50℃. Sterilize HT stock solution with membrane filtration and store solution in 2 - 5 mL aliquots at - 20℃. The hypoxanthine might precipitate out of solution during storage. Re-dissolve them by heating in a boiling water bath.

(2) 100 - fold concentrated stock solution of aminopterin (A): add 1.76 mg aminopterin (molecular weight 440.4 Da) to 90 mL of twice-distilled water. Add 1 mol/L NaOH dropwise until the aminopterin dissolves and then titrate to pH 7.5 with 1 mol/L HCl. Adjust final volume to 100 mL with twice-distilled water. Sterilize stock solution A by membrane filtration, dispense into 2 - 5 mL aliquots and store them at −20℃.

5. HAT medium: add 2 mL of HT and 2 mL of A stock solutions to 96 mL of tissue culture medium containing 10% serum.

(Zhang Xiaolian)

附录二   实验常用小鼠的品系及模型

1. 常用小鼠的品系

品 系	缩写	毛 色	MHC II类基因的单体型	注 释
A/J	A	白 色	k	
AKR	AK	白 色	k	
BALB/C	C	白 色	d	多数患骨髓瘤的亲代为异基因
iCBA	CB	野鼠色	k	
C3H	C3	野鼠色	k	
C57BL/6	B6	黑 色	b	常用做转基因 F_2 的亲代
C57BL/10	B10	黑 色	b	多数 H_2 是同基因
DBA/2		淡褐色	d	常用做转基因 F_2 的亲代
NZB		黑 色	d	适合制作抗自身抗体
SJL		白 色	s	常用做转基因 F_2 的亲代
129		白色或浅银灰色	b	许多畸胎瘤的后代

2. 常用免疫缺陷鼠系

名 称	背 景	侵袭细胞
重症联合免疫缺陷(SCID)	CB.17	T 细胞,B 细胞
裸鼠(nu/nu)	BALB/c, C57BL/6,其他	T 细胞
Motheaten(me/me)	C57BL/6	T 细胞,B 细胞,非淋巴类细胞
Beige	C57BL/6	NK, PMN
显性斑	C57BL/6	干细胞
无毛	C3H	表皮细胞,免疫细胞

3. 常用自身免疫病小鼠模型鼠系

名 称	背 景	侵袭细胞
系统性自身免疫 NZB 模型	NZB(复合,多基因)	BMD
系统性自身免疫病 NZB×NZW F1 模型	NZB×NZW F1(复合,多基因)	
全身性淋巴腺病	C3H,其他	T 细胞,其他
NOD	ICR/Clea	

4. 常用的自身免疫性疾病转基因小鼠模型鼠系

转基因的表达	背　　景
抗红细胞抗体	C57BL/6
抗 DNA 抗体	C57BL/6
抗 H-2Kk 抗体	BALB/c
抗 H-Y TCR-α β	C57BL/6
抗 TLb TCR-γ δ	CBA/J×C57BL/6

（高劲松）

Appendice 2 Strains and Models of Mice Commonly Used in Experiments

1. Mouse Strains commonly used in lab experiments

Strains	Abbreviations	Coat color	Haplotype of MHC II genes	Notes
A/J	A	White	k	
AKR	AK	White	k	
BALB/C	C	White	d	Most of the parents who suffer from myeloma are heterogenic
iCBA	CB	Rat color	k	
C3H	C3	Rat color	k	
C57BL/6	B6	Black	b	Ofen used as parents of transgenic F_2
C57BL/10	B10	Black	b	Most H_2 is the same gene
DBA/2		Hazel	d	Ofen used as parents of transgenic F_2
NZB		Black	d	Suitable for preparing anti-auto antibodies
SJL		White	s	Ofen used as parents of transgenic F_2
129		Whiteorlight silver grey	b	Offspring of many teratomas

2. Mouse strains commonly used for immunodeficiency diseases

Name	Background	Invasive cell
SCID	CB.17	T cell, B cell
Nude mice(nu/nu)	BALB/c, C57BL/6, the others	T cell
Motheaten(me/me)	C57BL/6	T cell, B cell, non-lymphoid cells
Beige	C57BL/6	NK, PMN
Dominant spot	C57BL/6	Stem cell
glabrous	C3H	Epidermic cell, immune cell

3. Mouse strains commonly used in autoimmune disease models

Name	Background	Invasive cell
NZB model of systemic autoimmune	NZB(complex, polygenes)	BMD
NZB×NZW F1 model of systemic autoimmune	NZB×NZW F1(complex, polygenes)	
Systemic lymphadenopathy	C3H, the others	T cell, the others
NOD	ICR/Clea	

4. Mouse strains commonly used in transgenic mouse models

Expression of transgenes	Background
Anti-RBC antibody	C57BL/6
Anti-DNA antibody	C57BL/6
Anti-H－2Kk antibody	BALB/c
Anti-H－Y TCR－α β antibody	C57BL/6
Anti-TLb TCR－γ δ antibody	CBA/J×C57BL/6

（Gao Jinsong）